WEIGHT WATCHERS
FREESTYLE
COOKBOOK

The Ultimate Guide To Weight Watchers Freestyle Program Include 7 Day Meal Plan to Guarantee Success.

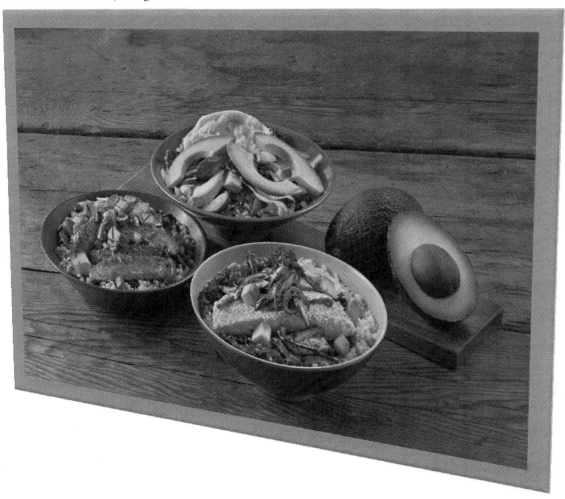

By Natasha Hayward

© Copyright 2019 by Natasha Hayward All rights reserved.
The following Book is reproduced below with the goal of providing information that is as accurate and as reliable as possible. Regardless, purchasing this Book can be seen as consent to the fact that both the publisher and the author of this book are in no way experts on the topics discussed within, and that any recommendations or suggestions made herein are for entertainment purposes only. Professionals should be consulted as needed before undertaking any of the action endorsed herein.

This declaration is deemed fair and valid by both the American Bar Association and the Committee of Publishers Association and is legally binding throughout the United States.

Furthermore, the transmission, duplication or reproduction of any of the following work, including precise information, will be considered an illegal act, irrespective whether it is done electronically or in print. The legality extends to creating a secondary or tertiary copy of the work or a recorded copy and is only allowed with express written consent of the Publisher. All additional rights are reserved.

The information in the following pages is broadly considered a truthful and accurate account of facts, and as such, any inattention, use or misuse of the information in question by the reader will render any resulting actions solely under their purview. There are no scenarios in which the publisher or the original author of this work can be in any fashion deemed liable for any hardship or damages that may befall them after undertaking information described herein.

Additionally, the information found on the following pages is intended for informational purposes only and should thus be considered, universal. As befitting its nature, the information presented is without assurance regarding its continued validity or interim quality. Trademarks that mentioned are done without written consent and can in no way be considered an endorsement from the trademark holder.

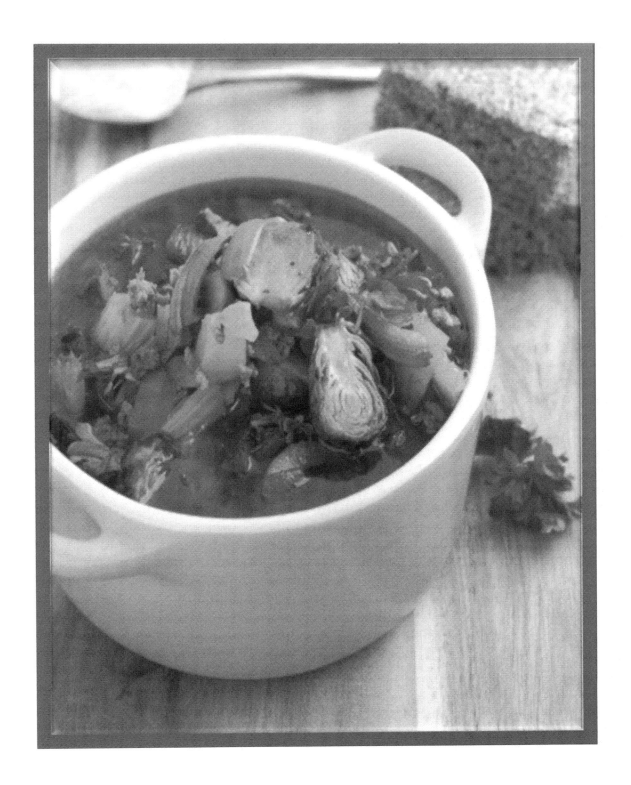

Table of Contents

Introduction 7
Weight Watchers 9
   The Change 9
   FreeStyle Program 14
   Total flexibility 15
   How It Works 15
   Rollover Points 15
   New Zero Points Food List 16
   200+ Zero Points Foods 17
   100 Most Tracked Foods With Smartpoints 23
Latest Freestyle Recipes 28
   oFS - Crock Pot Chicken Cacciatore 28
   oFS - Simple Garden Vegetable Soup 29
   oFS - Slow Cooker Shredded Chicken 31
   oFS - Beef Veggie Lentil Soup 31
   oFS - Succotash Bean Soup 32
   oFS - Beef Veggie Lentil Soup 33
   oFS – GreekStyle Chickpea Salad 35
   oFS - Zero Points Bean Soup: 36
   oFS - Grilled Lime Shrimp Kebabs 36
   oFS - Turkey Veggie Soup 37
   oFS - Chicken Enchilada Stuffed Zucchini 38
   oFS - Turkey Pumpkin Chili 40
   oFS - Slow Cooker Black Beans 41
   oFS - Crock Pot Chicken Taco Chili 41
   oFS - Authentic Shoyu Ahi Poke 43
   oFS - Red Pepper Muffin Tin Eggs 43
   oFS - Slow Cooked Chicken Verde 45
   oFS - Crockpot Tomato Balsamic Chicken 45
   oFS - Slow Cook Chicken Cacciatore 46
   oFS - Succotash Bean Soup 47
   1FS - Healthy Tuna Salad Wraps 47
   1FS - Cheesy Veggie Egg Scramble 48
   1FS - White Bean Turkey Chili 49
   1FS - Sweet & Sour Meatballs 50
   5FSP - Raspberry Chicken Salad 52
   5FS - Asparagus and Chicken Salad 52
   4FS - Simple Taco Salad 53
   4FS - Chicken and Spinach Rings 54
   5FS - Chicken Club Salad 55
   6FS - Roasted Caprese Salad Chicken 55
   5FS - Fresh Egg Salad 56

4FS - Fruit & Blue Cheese Tossed Salad ... 57
7FS - Sweet Potato Chili ... 58
6FS - Roasted Cauliflower Soup ... 59
5FS - Mushroom Egg Drop Soup ... 60
5FS - Tasty Turkey Meatball & Veggie ... 62
5FS - Creamy-Tomato-Basil-Soup ... 63
1FS - Chicken Taco Soup Recipe ... 63
5FS - Sticky Buffalo Chicken Tenders ... 64
5FS - Garlic Roasted Garbanzo Beans ... 65
1FS - Sweet & Sour Turkey Meatballs ... 66
5FS - Roasted Sweet Potato Side Dish ... 67
7FS - Apple Cheddar Turkey Wraps ... 67
2FS - Tasty BBQ Apricot Chicken ... 68
7FS - Pizza Lasagna Roll-Ups ... 69
3FS - Savory Chicken Dump Soup ... 70
5FS - Chicken Marsala MeatBall ... 71
4FS - Bruschetta Topped Balsamic Chicken ... 72
5FS - Ham & Apricot Dijon Glaze ... 74

7 Day Meal Plan ... 74

Let's Start ... 74

Monday ... 74
Tuesday ... 75
Wednesday ... 76
Thursday ... 77
Friday ... 78
Saturday ... 79
Sunday ... 79

WW Smart Points Main course Recipes ... 81

Honey Sesame Chicken ... 82
Chicken Fried Rice ... 82
Tasty Orange Chicken ... 83
Chicken and Sweet Potato ... 84
Beef Soba Bowls ... 85
Baked Artichoke Chicken ... 86
Garlic Thai Chicken ... 86
Pork Tenderloin with Broccoli ... 87
Easy Pork Piccata ... 88
Tender Spiced Pulled Pork ... 89
Curried Pork Chops ... 90
Spicy Pineapple Pork ... 91
Breaded Veal Cutlets ... 91
Cheesy Fajita Casserole ... 92
Spiced Pork with Apples ... 93

Pork Chops with Salsa 94
Italian Steak Rolls 95
Creamy Dijon Chicken 96
Light Chicken Salad 96
Turkey Mac with Jalapenos 97
Grilled Chicken Salad 98
Delicious Chicken Salad 98
Raspberry Balsamic Chicken 99

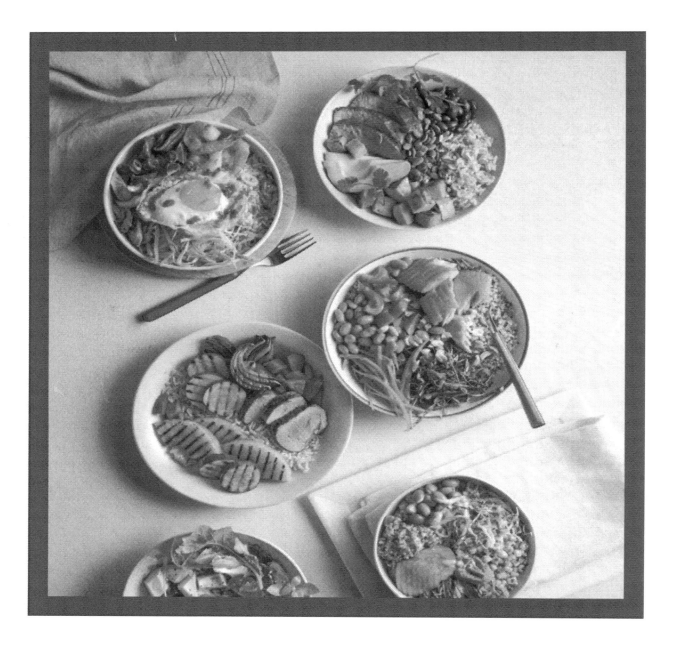

Introduction

The reasons why people lose weight vary from person to person. Over the past two decades, obesity has greatly increased in the USA with statistics showing that more than a third of adults in the USA are overweight. When one is overweight, he or she has a lot of physiological as well as emotional issues, hence people having varied reasons for wanting to lose weight:

- ***Being Healthy***

During a research carried out in 2007, half of the target population said their major reason for losing weight was to improve their health. When obese, one is at a risk of developing heart disease, stroke as well as cancer.

- ***Mood***

Why is this so? When one is overweight, he or she has insecurities that lead to depression as well as low self-esteem. Moreover, there is also some evidence that disorders related to one's mood and obesity is connected. Also, depression and bipolar disorder may be a precursor to obesity. Past studies have also proved that losing weight leads to improved mood.

- ***Fitness***

This is true especially for men who are regarded as being overweight.

- ***Wanting to have children***

This is because being overweight can lead to infertility and other complications during pregnancy. As we delve further into weight loss, the amount of weight you need to shed isn't really an important thing as such. You really need to know your real reasons for wanting to lose weight. We may have several reasons for wanting to shed weight, but we may not really realize what they are. When people are asked why they need to lose weight, most of them say: they want to be fit and healthy, they want to be confident, respected, love and so forth.

Consequently, you may start feeling trapped by your weight. You will start being obsessed about what you eat and the amount of exercise you do. There may be people who are leaner than you, but they are less confident, feel less loved and respected. Please be careful to lose weight for the correct reasons. If you have some solid reason for losing weight, you will definitely stick to your diet plan. There are good reasons as well as bad reasons for losing weight. The bad reasons may make you lose weight, but they will not be good enough for a long-term change in one's habits and lifestyle.

Good reasons for losing weight revolve around you while the negative ones revolve around pleasing other people such as:

- Shedding weight so as to attract someone

This may be a great trigger for weight loss; looking nice for someone you would want to be with. However, ask yourself what happens if this person does not exist in your life anymore? You will definitely lose your motivation for losing weight.

- Weight loss to boost health

This will be about you and it does not depend on what someone else thinks, says or does.

- Being referred to as overweight

Insults could motivate you to change your appearance. However, you don't need to change so as to impress someone.

In short, losing weight needs to be about you and nobody else. This is the only way to maintain your motivation and be focused on your goals.

Many people, including you, who is reading this, don't understand the main reasons why they want to lose weight. Your reasons for weight loss should be deeper and meaningful; they need to originate from your inner self. As soon as you have your valid reasons for losing weight, jot them down on an index card. Place them by your bedside and read them when you wake up and before retiring to bed.

Furthermore, you can also keep a copy at work and another in your wallet as a constant reminder of your goals.

You should also know that weight-loss goals, determine the difference between success and failure. Goals that are well-planned will keep you focused and motivated. Goals that are not realistic and overly ambitious will definitely undermine your efforts. Below are tips on losing weight:

- Concentrate on process goals

An outcome goal could be what you hope to achieve in the end. Even though this goal may give you a target, it does not guide you on how to achieve it. A process goal is a vital step in achieving whatever you desire. For instance, a process goal could be eating five portions of fruits or veggies on a daily basis, walking for half an hour daily or maybe drinking water after every meal. Process goals are particularly helpful when losing weight because you will focus on changing behaviors and habits that are important in weight loss.

- Set smart goals
1. They need to be specific- a good goal needs to have specific details.
2. They need to be measurable- if you can measure a goal, then you can objectively determine how successful you are at achieving the goal.
3. They need to be achievable- For instance, if your schedule doesn't allow you to spend an hour at the gym, then this is an unattainable goal.
4. They need to be realistic
- Your goals also need to be track-able
- Have long-term and short-term goals
- Don't try to be perfect

Setbacks are a natural part of behavior change. No one who is successful has never experienced setbacks. Identify potential barriers.

- Reassess and adjust goals as required

Weight Watchers

The Change

People used to strive for ways to find food. As the world advanced, we have so much of food that we don't know how to stop consuming it. That's where diet programs come in. The market is now congested with different dietary programs, all making claims of being the best. But few have achieved the heights that Weight Watchers has. And to know the secret behind Weight Watchers success we take an in-depth look into what makes it stand out.

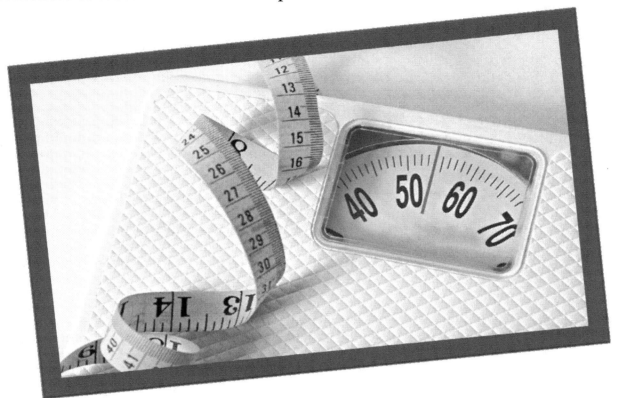

We human beings live of motivation, without it we do not go far. Our surroundings play a vital role in that. That's what makes Weight Watchers so keen on providing you with the perfect community. People whom you can get motivated from and whom you motivate. People from different walks of life come into meetings where they share their successes and their failures providing them with the perfect encouragement to carry on with their diets. So often many of us do not have either the time or the right people around us to support us when we stand on the scale and feel broken by the number we see displayed. The community and its active meetings provide the perfect antidote for all these mental challenges that every overweight man and woman faces.

Evolution is what has kept us human beings the dominating creature. And this precise idea is what Weight Watchers have used to keep them on top. Weight Watchers introduces new and different ways to deal with so many of our daily problems. People who cannot attend meetings for any certain reasons can make use of the online forums, message boards and support groups. The newly introduced point system is also an example of how easy they make dieting for people who do not have time to calculate every single calorie they are consuming. The website itself is a dieter's heaven having everything an honest dieter would need to keep him in check and informed.

Weight Watchers is a great dieting program that is going to help you to lose weight in a safe and effective way. While other diet programs focus on really limiting your calories and telling you what you are allowed to eat and what you should stay away from. While this may work for some people, it can be a big challenge to always be kept away from some of their favourite foods. Plus making food purchases can be difficult on some of the diet plans.

Weight Watchers is going to work a bit differently. It realizes that you have a lot going on in life and you won't be able to sit around and purchase expensive products or go after hard to find ingredients in order to stay healthy. This one is based on the Smart Points that will allow you to eat the foods that work the best for you, but it does reward the healthy foods and discourages the unhealthy foods.

This plan is all about being conscious about your personal eating choices. You will be given a certain amount of points that you are able to use each day, and you get to choose how you use them up. Each of the foods that you choose will have a different point value assigned to it, and you can even make your own recipes and figure out the point values.

This program does allow you to have a bit of cheating throughout the week if you are really craving it or you are not able to resist for a big party. You will find that you can place these into your points values for the day and still eat them. As long as you are smart about some of the choices that you are making for the rest of the day, these little cheats are not going to ruin the hard work that you put in.

In addition to worrying about the healthy foods that you should consume during the week, there are other parts that come with Weight Watchers. These include going to the meetings and getting more activity into your daily life.

Acknowledging the fact that exercise is a very primal factor in having a fit body is one of the positive points of Weight Watchers too. The program changes the way people perceive health from only being related to what you eat to being related to what you exercise as well. The program also works at changing how people think about health and food in general. Making them aware of the rights and wrongs of their daily routines.

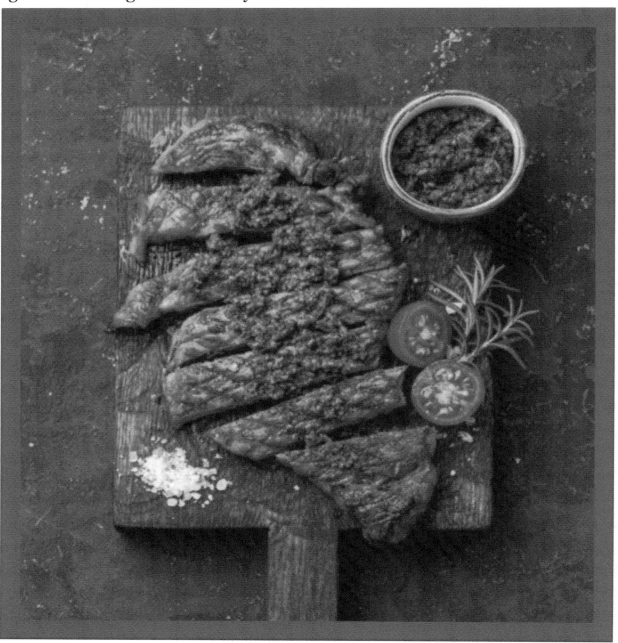

Eating on Weight Watchers is easier than you are going to find on many of the other diet plans. While these other diet plans tell you exactly what you can eat and what you should avoid, Weight Watchers takes a slightly different approach. They don't expressly tell you that you can't have any type of food because they know that life happens. They know that you aren't going to make it through the holidays without having some treats and they know that sometimes you just have a bad day and need to cheat a bit.

This is a normal life. We all have those times when it is just too hard to stay on a diet plan, and we need something that is not all that healthy for us. And this is why Weight Watchers doesn't forbid any type of food like the other diet plans; it simply gives us the tools that we need to make healthy choices. We are allowed to have that cookie on occasion, and it will fit into our points, as long as we made other healthy choices along the way.

Why Choose Weight Watchers?

There are a lot of great diet plans that you can choose to go with. Some are going to choose to have you limit your carb intake while others are going to limit the fats. Some are healthy while others are going to be hard to maintain because they are so hard on the body. Weight Watchers is a bit different than all of these because you get some options. Some of the reasons that you should choose to go with Weight Watchers instead of another weight loss program includes:

- Lose more weight—overall, people who go on a program similar to Weight Watchers are able to lose more weight than with other options. This is because it is flexible to follow and you have that motivation and support going to the meetings each week.
- Flexibility—there is a lot of flexibility that comes with being on Weight Watchers. You get to enjoy the ability to pick the foods that you want to consume, when you want to eat them and even how much, based on the amount of points that you are allowed. You can also pick your activity levels, your meetings, whether to have the meetings in person or online and so much more! This makes it easier for everyone to find the path on this plan that works best for them.

- Lifestyle change—Weight Watchers is not just about losing weight. It is about making changes in your whole lifestyle that will result in healthy weight loss. You are going to learn how to eat foods that are healthier and full of nutrition while getting rid of the foods that are causing weight gain and health issues. You are going to learn how important activity is in your life and start to implement it in more. You will work on getting healthier stress levels and sleeping as well.
- Eat the foods you like—you are the one in charge of the foods that you eat on this diet plan, so you can eat some of your favourites as well. While you do need to make some healthier choices when it comes to staying within your points, there is still the option of having some of your favourite meals on occasion.
- Ability to fit it into your daily life—it is possible to fit this diet plan into your daily life. You are able to eat real foods, foods that taste good, and will fill you up. You can choose to work out each day or do normal activities, such as chores, around the house, without having to spend hours at the gym each day. The foods can be your normal favourites as long as you are careful about not eating too much.
- You can eat out—when you are on this plan, you are allowed to eat out. While you shouldn't do this each day, eating out every once in a while is not a sin of this diet plan. It realizes that there are times you will go out with friends and family and realizing that you can go out as long as you make the right decisions for the rest of the day and don't overdo it with eating at the restaurant, you will be fine without ruining all your hard work.
- People to help you along the way—there are weekly meetings that you can attend that will help you to stay on your plan. You can meet with others who will motivate you along your journey and will help you any time that things get tuff or you need some help. It is hard to find this kind of motivation on the other diet plans that you pick.

There is no diet plan that is the same as Weight Watchers for all the flexibility and support that you are going to get along the way. If you have been trying to lose weight in the past and are ready to take that step to seeing a lot of success finally, make sure to check out Weight Watchers and see how it can work for you.

FreeStyle Program

Based on the successful SmartPoints® system, WW Freestyle offers more than 200 zero Points® foods—including eggs, skinless chicken breast, fish and seafood, corn, beans, peas, and so much more—to multiply your meal and menu possibilities. And it makes life simpler, too: You can forget about weighing, measuring, or tracking those zero Points foods.

Total flexibility

And because we recognize that every day is different—and some days are *really* different (think parties, business travel, holiday open houses....)—we've made your SmartPoints Budget more flexible than ever. Up to 4 unused daily SmartPoints can now roll over into your weekly SmartPoints to give you a bigger "bank" to use whenever and however you like.

How It Works

- For those of you not already familiar with SmartPoints, the SmartPoints system uses the latest nutritional science to make healthy eating as simple as possible. It nudges you toward making healthy choices so eat better and lose weight.
- Every food and drink has a SmartPoints value: a number that is based on calories, protein, sugar and saturated fat. The baseline SmartPoints value is based on the food's calories. Protein lowers the SmartPoints value. Saturated fat and sugar increase the SmartPoints value.
- Every day you get a SmartPoints Budget to spend on any foods you want.
- Your Daily SmartPoints Budget is calculated based on your age, height, weight and gender with a minimum daily value of 23.
- You only need to track the foods that have a SmartPoints value.
- You don't need to weigh, measure or track 0 SmartPoints foods.
- Enjoy a greatly total list of 0 SmartPoints go-to foods at the end of this book.
- Every week you also get a Weekly SmartPoints Budget that you can think of as "overdraft" protection. They are there to use when you go over your Daily SmartPoints budget.
- You can roll over up to four (4) unused Daily SmartPoints into your Weekly SmartPoints. Use them or not as you see fit.

Rollover Points

With the new Weight Watchers Freestyle plan for 2018, you will be able to roll over up to 4 SmartPoints daily if you do not use them.

I love this idea since it means you could adjust your points to match the natural rhythms and fluctuations of your appetite.

Here are some of the latest recipes available so you can try out the Freestyle program

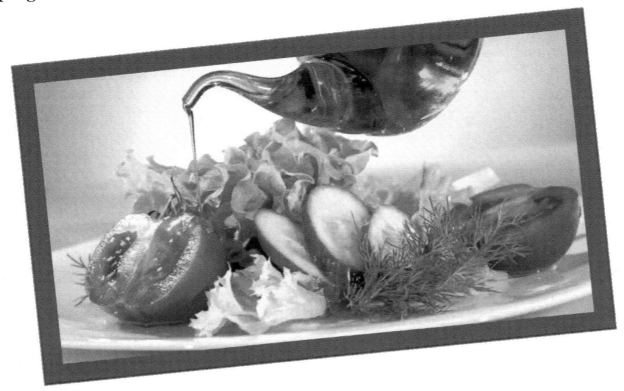

New Zero Points Food List

Zero Point Foods

Instead of counting calories, Weight Watchers uses a point system to help control what you eat to lose weight. A mathematical equation focused on saturated fat, sugar, carb and calorie content is used to determine the point value for a food. Zero point foods are low in all these categories. All fresh fruit and most vegetables have zero points, with the exception of starchy vegetables such as corn or potatoes. In addition to helping fill you up without costing you any points, the list is used to help dieters on the Weight Watchers program make healthier food choices.

-

Nonstarchy Veggies

People who eat more vegetables tend to weigh less. Veggies are low in calories and high in fiber, so they fill you up without making too much of an impact on your calorie intake. Any nonstarchy vegetable is a zero point food. These include broccoli, cauliflower, carrots, cucumbers, peppers, onions, snow peas, zucchini, greens and lettuce. When you feel a little hungry while following the Weight Watchers diet, you can make yourself a salad and enjoy it without having to worry about points.

All Kinds of Fruit

As with veggies, eating more fruit might help you weigh less. Although not as low in calories as nonstarchy vegetables, fruit is still lower in calories than a cookie or an ice cream cone, and it's more nutritious too. Any fresh fruit, even those banned from other diets such as grapes and bananas, have zero points on the Weight Watchers plan. Apples, oranges, strawberries, kiwi, watermelon and pears have zero points. Eating these healthy foods satisfies your taste buds and your appetite. Add sliced strawberries to your zero point salad for a touch of sweetness.

Food Flavorings and Special Treats

You can flavor your food without feeling guilty with a number of different items on the zero point list, such as vinegar, lemon or lime juice, hot sauce, ketchup, mustard, salsa and soy sauce. Drizzle a little vinegar on your salad to complete your zero point snack.

Broth, which you can sip on a cold day to keep you warm and satisfy your craving for something savory, is also a zero point food. You can consume sugar-free ice pops, diet soda and sugar-free gelatin without sacrificing any of your points as well.

200+ Zero Points Foods

Here it is: an expanded list of all 200+ zero Points foods. The foods on this list form the foundation of a healthy eating pattern, so you don't need to weigh, measure, or track any of them

- Apples
- Applesauce, unsweetened
- Apricots
- Arrowroot
- Artichoke hearts
- Artichokes
- Arugula
- Asparagus

- Bamboo shoots
- Banana
- Beans: including adzuki, black, broad (fava), butter, cannellini, cranberry (Roman), green, garbanzo (chickpeas), great northern, kidney, lima, lupini, mung, navy, pink, pinto, small white, snap, soy, string, wax, white
- Beans, refried, fat-free, canned
- Beets
- Berries, mixed
- Blackberries
- Blueberries
- Broccoli
- Broccoli rabe
- Broccoli slaw
- Broccolini
- Brussels sprouts

- Cabbage: all varieties including Chinese (bok choy), Japanese, green, red, napa, savory, pickled
- Calamari, grilled
- Cantaloupe
- Carrots
- Cauliflower
- Caviar
- Celery
- Swiss chard

- Cherries
- Chicken breast, ground, 99% fat-free
- Chicken breast or tenderloin, skinless, boneless or with bone
- Clementines
- Coleslaw mix (shredded cabbage and carrots), packaged
- Collards
- Corn, baby (ears), white, yellow, kernels, on the cob
- Cranberries
- Cucumber

- Daikon
- Dates, fresh
- Dragon fruit

- Edamame, in pods or shelled
- Egg substitutes
- Egg whites
- Eggplant
- Eggs, whole, including yolks
- Endive
- Escarole

- Fennel (anise, sweet anise, or finocchio)
- Figs
- Fish: anchovies, arctic char, bluefish, branzino (sea bass), butterfish, carp, catfish, cod, drum, eel, flounder, grouper, haddock, halibut, herring, mackerel, mahimahi (dolphinfish), monkfish, orange roughy, perch, pike, pollack, pompano, rainbow trout (steelhead), rockfish, roe, sablefish (including smoked), salmon (all varieties), salmon, smoked (lox), sardines, sea bass, smelt, snapper, sole, striped bass, striped mullet, sturgeon (including smoked); white sucker, sunfish (pumpkinseed), swordfish, tilapia, tilefish, tuna (all varieties), turbot, whitefish (including smoked), whitefish and pike (store-bought), whiting
- Fish fillet, grilled with lemon pepper
- Fruit cocktail
- Fruit cup, unsweetened
- Fruit salad

- Fruit, unsweetened

- Garlic
- Ginger root
- Grapefruit
- Grapes
- Greens: beet, collard, dandelion, kale, mustard, turnip
- Greens, mixed baby
- Guavas
- Guavas, strawberry

- Hearts of palm (palmetto)
- Honeydew melon
- Jackfruit
- Jerk chicken breast
- Jerusalem artichokes (sunchokes)
- Jicama (yam bean)

- Kiwifruit
- Kohlrabi
- Kumquats

- Leeks
- Lemon
- Lemon zest
- Lentils
- Lettuce, all varieties
- Lime
- Lime zest
- Litchis (lychees)

- Mangoes
- Melon balls
- Mung bean sprouts
- Mung dal
- Mushroom caps

- Mushrooms: all varieties including brown, button, crimini, Italian, portabella, shiitake

- Nectarine
- Nori seaweed

- Okra
- Onions
- Oranges: all varieties including blood

- Papayas
- Parsley
- Passion fruit
- Pea shoots
- Peaches
- Peapods, black-eye
- Pears
- Peas and carrots
- Peas: black-eyed, chickpeas (garbanzo), cowpeas (blackeyes, crowder, southern), young pods with seeds, green, pigeon, snow (Chinese pea pods); split, sugar snap
- Peppers, all varieties
- Pepperoncini
- Persimmons
- Pickles, unsweetened
- Pico de gallo
- Pimientos, canned
- Pineapple
- Plumcots (pluots)
- Plums
- Pomegranate seeds
- Pomegranates
- Pomelo (pummelo)
- Pumpkin
- Pumpkin puree

- Radicchio

- Radishes
- Raspberries
- Rutabagas

- Salad, mixed greens
- Salad, side, without dressing, fast food
- Salad, three-bean
- Salad, tossed, without dressing
- Salsa verde
- Salsa, fat free
- Salsa, fat free; gluten-free
- Sashimi
- Satay, chicken, without peanut sauce
- Satsuma mandarin
- Sauerkraut
- Scallions
- Seaweed
- Shallots
- Shellfish: abalone, clams, crab (including Alaska king, blue, dungeness, lump crabmeat, queen) crayfish, cuttlefish, lobster (including spiny lobster), mussels, octopus, oysters, scallops, shrimp, squid
- Spinach
- Sprouts, including alfalfa, bean, lentil
- Squash, summer (all varieties including zucchini)
- Squash, winter (all varieties including spaghetti)
- Starfruit (carambola)
- Strawberries
- Succotash

- Tangelo
- Tangerine
- Taro
- Tofu, all varieties
- Tofu, smoked
- Tomatillos
- Tomato puree
- Tomato sauce

- Tomatoes: all varieties including plum, grape, cherry
- Turkey breast, ground, 99% fat-free
- Turkey breast or tenderloin, skinless, boneless or with bone
- Turkey breast, skinless, smoked
- Turnips

- Vegetable sticks
- Vegetables, mixed
- Vegetables, stir fry, without sauce

- Water chestnuts
- Watercress
- Watermelon

- Yogurt, Greek, plain, nonfat, unsweetened
- Yogurt, plain, nonfat, unsweetened
- Yogurt, soy, plain

---

100 Most Tracked Foods With Smartpoints

	Name	Amount	Points
1	Almond milk, plain, unsweetened	1 cup	1
2	Almonds	1/4 cup	4
3	American cheese	1 slice or 1 ounce	4
4	Apple		0
5	Asparagus		0
6	Avocado, Hass	1/4	2
7	Bacon, cooked	3 slices	5
8	Bagel, any type	1 small or 1/2 large, 2 ounces	5
9	Banana		0
10	Beef, ground, 90% lean, cooked	3 ounces	4
11	Beer, regular	12 ounces	5
12	Berries, mixed		0
13	Black beans, canned	1/2 cup	3
14	Blackberries		0
15	Blueberries		0
16	Bread	1 slice	2
17	Broccoli		0
18	Brown rice, cooked	1 cup	6
19	Butter	1 tablespoon	5
20	Cantaloupe		0
21	Carrots		0
22	Carrots, baby		0
23	Celery		0
24	Cheddar cheese, shredded	1/4 cup	4
25	Cheddar or Colby cheese	1 ounce	4
26	Cherries		0

27	Cherry tomatoes		0
28	Chicken breast, cooked, boneless, skinless	3 ounces	2
29	Coffee, black, without sugar	1 cup	0
30	Cookies, homemade, chocolate, chip, oatmeal, sugar or similar type	1 or 1/2 ounce	3
31	Corn on the cob	1 medium	4
32	Cottage cheese, fat-free	1 cup	2
33	Cream, half and half	2 tablespoons	2
34	Cucumber		0
35	Deli sliced turkey	2 ounces	1
36	Diet Coke	8 ounces	0
37	Egg white	1	0
38	Egg	1	2
39	Egg, fried	1	3
40	Eggs scrambled with milk and butter	2 or 1/2 cup	6
41	English muffin	1 or 2 ounces	4
42	Feta, crumbled	1 ounce	3
43	French fries	20 or 5.5 ounces	13
44	Fruit, fresh, unsweetened		0
45	Grape tomatoes		0
46	Grapefruit		0
47	Grapes		0
48	Green beans		0
49	Guacamole	2 tablespoons	1
50	Half and half, fat-free	2 tablespoons	1

51	Hamburger bun, plain	1 or 2 ounces	5
52	Honey	1 tablespoon	4
53	Hummus	2 tablespoons	2
54	Lettuce		0
55	Luncheon meat, ham, honey, lean, deli-sliced	2 ounces	2
56	Mango		0
57	Mashed potatoes	1/2 cup	4
58	Mayonnaise	1 tablespoon	3
59	Milk, low fat 1%	1 cup	4
60	Milk, reduced fat 2%	1 cup	5
61	Milk, skim (fat-free)	1 cup	3
62	Milk, whole	1 cup	7
63	Mushrooms		0
64	Mustard	1 tablespoon	0
65	Nectarine		0
66	Oatmeal, cooked	1 cup	5
67	Olive oil	1 tablespoon	4
68	Onions		0
69	Orange		0
70	Pasta, regular or whole wheat, cooked,	1 cup	5
71	Peach		0
72	Peanut butter	2 tablespoons	6
73	Pear		0
74	Pineapple		0
75	Pork chop, cooked, lean, boneless	3 ounces	3
76	Potato, baked, plain	1, 6 ounces	5

#	Item	Serving	Points
77	Raspberries		0
78	Red wine	5 ounces	4
79	Salad dressing, balsamic vinaigrette, low-fat	1 tablespoons	1
80	Salad dressing, Italian-type (not creamy)	2 tablespoons	3
81	Salad dressing, ranch	2 tablespoons	5
82	Salad, mixed greens		0
83	Salsa, fat-free		0
84	Shrimp, cooked	3 ounces	1
85	Spinach		0
86	Strawberries		0
87	Sugar, white, granulated	1 teaspoon	1
88	Sweet Potatoes, cooked	1/2 cup	3
89	Sweet red peppers		0
90	Tomatoes		0
91	Tortilla chips	1 ounce	4
92	Tortilla, flour	1 medium or 1 ounce	3
93	Tuna fish, canned in water, drained	3 ounces	1
94	Turkey bacon, cooked	3 slices	3
95	Water		0
96	Watermelon		0
97	White rice, cooked	1 cup	6
98	White wine	5 ounces	4
99	Yogurt, Greek, plain, fat-free	1 cup	3
100	Zucchini		0

Latest Freestyle Recipes

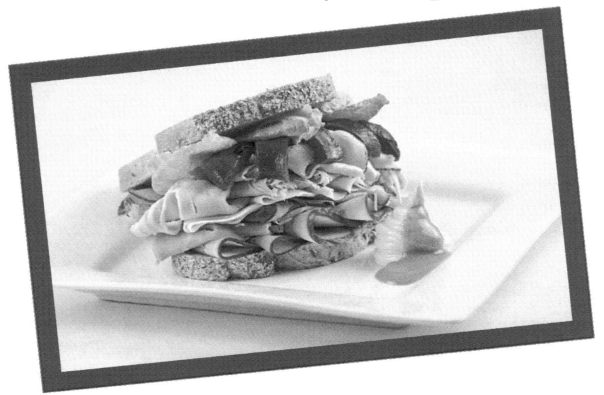

0FS - Crock Pot Chicken Cacciatore

(Prep time:10 min | Cook time:10 min | Total time:20 min | Serves: 5)

INGREDIENTS:
- 8 bone-in, skinless chicken thighs (about 5-ounces each), fat trimmed- in the photos for this recipe, you'll notice that I actually used 5 full chicken legs (drumstick and thigh) instead
- 3/4 teaspoon kosher salt
- freshly ground black pepper
- cooking spray
- 5 garlic cloves, finely chopped
- 1/2 large onion, chopped
- 1 28-ounce can crushed tomatoes
- 1/2 medium red bell pepper, chopped
- 1/2 medium green bell pepper, chopped

- 4 ounce sliced shiitake mushrooms
- 1 sprig of fresh thyme
- 1 sprig of fresh oregano
- 1 bay leaf
- 1 tablespoon chopped fresh parsley (I omitted this)
- freshly grated Parmesan cheese, for serving (optional)

DIRECTIONS:
1. Season the chicken with salt and pepper to taste. Heat a large nonstick skillet over medium-high heat. Coat with cooking spray, add the chicken, and cook until browned- 2 to 3 minutes per side. Transfer to your slow cooker.
2. Reduce the heat under the skillet to medium and coat with more cooking spray. Add the garlic and onion and cook, stirring, until soft- 3 to 4 minutes.
3. Transfer to the slow cooker and add the tomatoes, bell peppers, mushrooms, thyme, oregano and bay leaf. Stir to combine.
4. Cover and cook on high for 4 hours or on low for 8 hours.
5. Discard the bay leaf and transfer the chicken to a large plate. Pull the chicken meat from the bones (discard the bones), shred the meat, and return it to the sauce.
6. Stir in the parsley (if using). If desired, serve topped with Parmesan cheese.

Nutritional information per serving: Calories: 220, Fat: 6g, Sat Fat: 1.5g, Cholesterol: 123mg, Sodium: 319mg, Carbohydrates: 10g, Fiber: 2g, Sugar: 6g, Protein: 31g

0 SmartPoints on FreeStyle Plan

0FS - Simple Garden Vegetable Soup

(Prep time:15 min | Cook time:30 min | Total time:45 min | Serves: 5)

Ingredients

- 1/2 cup chopped onion
- 1/2 cup chopped carrots
- 1/2 cup chopped celery
- 2 garlic cloves, pressed
- 4 cups fat-free broth of your choice

- 1 can (14-1/2 ounces) diced tomatoes
- 1 cup chopped cabbage
- 1 cup chopped spinach or kale
- 1 tablespoon tomato paste
- 1/2 teaspoon dried basil (or more to taste)
- 1/2 teaspoon dried thyme (or more to taste)
- 1/2 teaspoon salt
- 1 cup chopped zucchini
- Chopped parsley or basil for garnish (optional)

Instructions

1. Spray a large saucepan or soup pot with nonstick cooking spray. Add the onion, carrot and celery and cook over low heat, stirring often until the vegetables have softened.
2. Add the garlic and stir for another minute.
3. Add the broth, tomatoes, cabbage, spinach, tomato paste, basil, thyme and salt and bring to a boil over medium high heat. Lower the heat, cover the pot and simmer gently for about 15 minutes.
4. Add the zucchini and cook until softened, 3 - 5 minutes more.
5. Stir in chopped fresh parsley or basil just before serving if desired.

Slow Cooker Instructions

1. Place everything in your slow cooker, cover and cook on LOW until tender, 6 to 8 hours.

Nutrition Facts
Amount per Serving (1 cup)
Calories 41Calories from Fat 8
0 SmartPoints on FreeStyle Plan

0FS - Slow Cooker Shredded Chicken

(Prep time:5 min | Cook time:4 h | Total time:6h 5 min | Serves: 3)

Ingredients
- 3-4 lbs. chicken breast, raw
- 4-5 cups low sodium chicken broth
- 3-4 tabs dried minced onion
- 1 tabs garlic powder
- 1 1/2 tsp celery salt
- 1 tsp pepper

Instructions
1. In a 6-quart slow cooker, add chicken breasts, broth, and seasonings.
2. Cook on low for 6 hours, or high for 4 hours.
3. Remove and transfer onto a cutting board, let cool, and shred into pieces. (Or shred with mixer)

Recipe Notes
Serving size: 3 oz.
0 SmartPoints on FreeStyle Plan

0FS - Beef Veggie Lentil Soup

(Prep time:10 min | Cook time:10 min | Total time:20 min | Serves: 5)

INGREDIENTS:
- 10 cups reduced-sodium beef broth
- 1 pound dried lentils, picked over, rinsed & drained
- 4 large carrots, peeled and finely chopped
- 1 large onion, peeled and finely chopped
- 2 large celery stalks, finely chopped
- 2 bay leaves
- One 14.5-ounce can diced tomatoes, with juice
- 1 tablespoon red wine vinegar
- freshly ground black pepper

- 1 to 2 cups hot water
- chopped chives for garnish, optional

DIRECTIONS:
1. In a large pot, combine the broth, lentils, carrots, onions, celery, and bay leaves; bring to a boil. Reduce the heat, and simmer, covered, stirring occasionally, until the lentils and vegetables are tender (about 30 minutes).
2. Add the tomatoes (with juice), vinegar and pepper. Add the water (amount depending on how much soupy broth you desire). Cover and cook, stirring occasionally, until the flavors have blended, 10 minutes.
3. Sprinkle individual servings with chives, if desired.

Nutritional Information per Serving (serving size 1 3/4 cups) Calories: 261, Fat: 2g, Saturated Fat: 0, Cholesterol: 0, Sodium: 364mg, Carbohydrates: 44g, Fiber 15g, Protein: 19g, Calcium: 72mg

0 SmartPoints on FreeStyle Plan

0FS - Succotash Bean Soup

(Prep time:10 min | Cook time:10 min | Total time:20 min | Serves: 5)

(12 approximately 1 cup servings)
Ingredients:

2 cans white beans (rinsed and drained)
2 cans Lima beans (rinsed and drained)
2 cans corn kernels drained
1 carton low sodium vegetable broth
12 slices Canadian bacon chopped into small pieces
Season to taste

Instructions
Dump all ingredients into a large crockpot. Stir gently to evenly mix ingredients. Cook on low 6-8 hours. This is zero points...you have enough left for cornbread!

0 SmartPoints on FreeStyle Plan

0FS - Beef Veggie Lentil Soup

(Prep time:10 min | Cook time:10 min | Total time:20 min | Serves: 5)

INGREDIENTS:
- 10 cups reduced-sodium beef broth
- 1 pound dried lentils, picked over, rinsed & drained
- 4 large carrots, peeled and finely chopped
- 1 large onion, peeled and finely chopped
- 2 large celery stalks, finely chopped
- 2 bay leaves
- One 14.5-ounce can diced tomatoes, with juice
- 1 tablespoon red wine vinegar
- freshly ground black pepper
- 1 to 2 cups hot water
- chopped chives for garnish, optional

DIRECTIONS:
4. In a large pot, combine the broth, lentils, carrots, onions, celery, and bay leaves; bring to a boil. Reduce the heat, and simmer, covered, stirring occasionally, until the lentils and vegetables are tender (about 30 minutes).
5. Add the tomatoes (with juice), vinegar and pepper. Add the water (amount depending on how much soupy broth you desire). Cover and cook, stirring occasionally, until the flavors have blended, 10 minutes.
6. Sprinkle individual servings with chives, if desired.

Nutritional Information per Serving (serving size 1 3/4 cups) Calories: 261, Fat: 2g, Saturated Fat: 0, Cholesterol: 0, Sodium: 364mg, Carbohydrates: 44g, Fiber 15g, Protein: 19g, Calcium: 72mg

0 SmartPoints on FreeStyle Plan

oFS - Mexican Chicken Soup

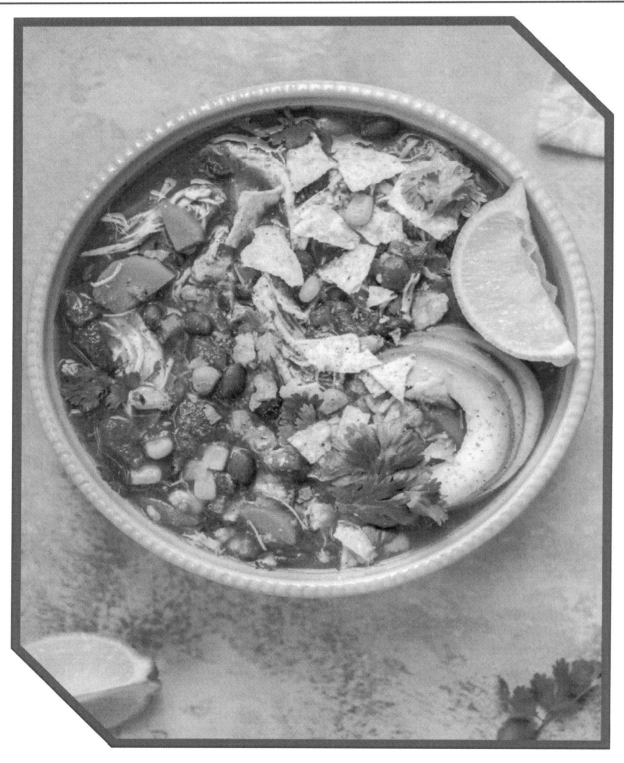

(Prep time:15 min | Cook time:6 H | Total time:6 H 15 min | Serves: 10)

Ingredients
- 2 cups salsa chicken shredded
- 1 small onion chopped
- 2 cloves garlic crushed
- 1 20 ounces can crushed tomatoes
- 1 12 ounces can great northern beans
- 1 12 ounces can red kidney beans
- 1 cup frozen whole kernel corn
- 6 cups fat-free chicken stock
- 1 tablespoon cumin
- 1 teaspoon garlic powder
- 1 teaspoon onion powder
- 1 teaspoon paprika
- 1 teaspoon chili powder
- 1 teaspoon black pepper
- 1 teaspoon salt

Instructions
1. Mix all ingredients together in large Crockpot.
2. Cook on low heat for 6 hours or high heat for 3 hours.
3. Serve alone or with tortilla chips or strips as desired.

0 SmartPoints on FreeStyle Plan

0FS – GreekStyle Chickpea Salad

0 WW Freestyle SP per serving.

INGREDIENTS
- 2 (15 ounce) cans chickpea, drained and rinsed
- 1 small tomato, chopped
- ¼ cup finely chopped red onion
- ½ teaspoon sugar
- ¼ cup reduced fat crumbled feta cheese
- ½ tablespoon lemon juice
- ½ tablespoon red wine vinegar
- 1 tablespoon plain nonfat Greek Yogurt
- 2 cloves garlic, minced
- ¼ teaspoon salt
- ¼ teaspoon pepper

- 1-2 tablespoons cilantro

INSTRUCTIONS
1. Drain and rinse the chickpeas and place in a medium bowl.
2. Toss in the rest of the ingredients until chickpeas are evenly coated and all of the ingredients are mixed well.
3. Serve immediately and refrigerate any leftovers.

Nutrition Information
- Serves: 8 servings
- Serving size: ½ cup
- Calories: 192
- Fat: 4 g
- Saturated fat: 1 g
- Carbohydrates: 32 g
- Sugar: 6 g
- Fiber: 8 g
- Protein: 10 g
- Cholesterol: 4 mg

0FS - Zero Points Bean Soup:

0 WW Freestyle Smart Points (12 approximately 1 cup servings)

Ingredients:
- 2 cans white beans (rinsed and drained)
- 2 cans Lima beans (rinsed and drained)
- 2 cans corn kernels drained
- 1 carton low sodium vegetable broth
- 12 slices Canadian Bacon chopped into small pieces
- Season to taste,

Directions:
1. Dump all ingredients into a large crockpot.
2. Stir gently to evenly mix ingredients.
3. Cook on low 6-8 hours. This is zero points…you have enough left for cornbread!

0FS - Grilled Lime Shrimp Kebabs

(Prep time:10 min | Cook time:20 min | Total time:30 min | Serves: 4)

INGREDIENTS:

- 32 jumbo raw shrimp, peeled and deveined (17.5 oz. after peeled)
- 3 cloves garlic, crushed
- 24 slices (about 3) large limes, very thinly sliced into rounds (optional)
- olive oil cooking spray (I use my mister)
- 1 tsp kosher salt
- 1 1/2 tsp ground cumin
- 1/4 cup chopped fresh cilantro, divided
- 16 bamboo skewers soaked in water 1 hour
- 1 lime cut into 8 wedges

DIRECTIONS:
1. Heat the grill on medium heat and spray the grates with oil.
2. Season the shrimp with garlic, cumin, salt and half of the cilantro in a medium bowl.
3. Beginning and ending with shrimp, thread the shrimp and folded lime slices onto 8 pairs of parallel skewers to make 8 kebabs total.
4. Grill the shrimp, turning occasionally, until shrimp is opaque throughout, about 1 to 2 minutes on each side.
5. Top with remaining cilantro and fresh squeezed lime juice before serving.

NUTRITION INFORMATION
Yield: 8 servings, Serving Size: 1 kebab
- **Amount Per Serving:**

Calories: 74, Total Fat: 1g, Saturated Fat: g
Carbohydrates: 3g, Fiber: 1g, Sugar: 0g, Protein: 13g

0 SmartPoints on FreeStyle Plan

0FS - Turkey Veggie Soup

(Prep time:20 min | Cook time:20 min | Total time:40 min | Serves: 6)
INGREDIENTS:
- 1 cup finely chopped celery (about 2 stalks)
- 1/2 cup finely chopped onion
- 1 1/2 teaspoons minced garlic
- 1 1/2 pounds 99% fat-free ground turkey breast
- 3 cups fat free beef or chicken broth
- 1 cup sliced carrot (about 2 large)

- 1/2 cup trimmed fresh green beans, cut in 1-inch lengths
- 1/2 cup frozen whole-kernel corn
- 1 1/2 teaspoons ground cumin
- 1 teaspoon chili powder
- 2 whole bay leaves
- One 15-ounce can kidney beans, rinsed and drained
- One 14.5-ounce can diced tomatoes and green chiles, undrained
- 6 tablespoons shredded Monterey Jack cheese, optional

DIRECTIONS:
1. Heat a Dutch oven over medium-high heat. Coat pan with cooking spray.
2. Add celery, onion, garlic and turkey. Cook 5 minutes or until ground turkey is browned, stirring to crumble. Add 3 cups of beef stock and remaining ingredients except cheese; bring to a boil. Cover, reduce heat, and simmer 20 minutes or until vegetables are tender. Discard bay leaves.
3. Ladle 1 1/2 cups soup into each of 6 bowls; top each serving with 1 Tablespoon of cheese.

Nutritional Information per serving: (Serving size: 1 1/2 cups soup- with 1 tablespoon of cheese) Calories: 265, Fat: 5g, Saturated Fat: 2g, Sugar: 7g, Sodium: 1789mg, Fiber: 7.5g, Protein: 27g, Cholesterol: 55mg, Carbohydrates per serving: 29g

0 SmartPoints on FreeStyle Plan

0FS - Chicken Enchilada Stuffed Zucchini

(Prep time:10 min | Cook time:10 min | Total time:20 min | Serves: 8)

Ingredients:
For the enchilada sauce:
- olive oil spray
- 2 garlic cloves, minced
- 1 or 2 tbsp. chipotle chile in adobo sauce, more if you like it spicy
- 1-1/2 cups tomato sauce
- 1/2 tsp chipotle chili powder
- 1/2 tsp ground cumin
- 2/3 cup fat-free low-sodium chicken broth

- kosher salt and fresh pepper to taste

For the zucchini boats:
- 4 (about 32 oz. total) medium zucchini
- 1 tsp oil
- 1/2 cup green onions, chopped
- 3 cloves garlic, crushed
- 1/2 cup diced green bell pepper
- 1/4 cup chopped cilantro
- 8 oz. cooked shredded chicken breast
- 1 tsp cumin
- 1/2 tsp dried oregano
- 1/2 tsp chipotle chili powder
- 3 tbsp. water or fat free chicken broth
- 1 tbsp. tomato paste
- salt and pepper to taste

For the Topping:
- 3/4 cup reduced fat shredded sharp cheddar
- chopped scallions and cilantro for garnish

Directions:

For the enchilada sauce: In a medium saucepan, **spray** oil and **sauté** garlic. **Add** chipotle chiles, chili powder, cumin, chicken broth, tomato sauce, salt and pepper. Bring to a boil. **Reduce** the heat to low and **simmer** for 5-10 minutes. Set aside until ready to use.

For the Zucchini Boats: Bring a large pot of water to boil. **Preheat** oven to 400°. **Cut** zucchini in half lengthwise and using a small spoon or melon baller, **scoop** out flesh, leaving 1/4" thick. **Chop** the scooped out flesh of the zucchini in small pieces and set aside.

Drop the zucchini halves in boiling water and cook 1 minute; **remove** from water.

In a large sauté pan, **heat** oil and **add** onion, garlic and bell pepper. **Cook** on medium-low heat for about 2-3 minutes, until onions are translucent. **Add** chopped zucchini and cilantro; **season** with salt and pepper and **cook** about 4 minutes. **Add** the cumin, oregano, chili powder, water, and tomato paste and cook a few more minutes, then **add** in chicken; **mix** and cook 3 more minutes.

Place 1/4 cup of the enchilada sauce on the bottom of a large (or 2 small) baking dish, and place zucchini halves cut side up. Using a spoon, **fill** each hollowed zucchini with 1/3 cup chicken mixture, pressing firmly.

Top each with 2 tablespoons of enchilada sauce, and 1 1/2 tablespoons each of shredded cheese.

Cover with foil and **bake** 35 minutes until cheese is melted and zucchini is cooked through.

Top with scallions and cilantro for garnish and serve with low fat sour cream if desired.

Servings: 8 • **Size:** 1 zucchini boat • **Calories:** 116 • **Fat:** 3.5 g • **Protein:** 12 g • **Carb:** 11 g • **Fiber:** 3 g • **Sugar:** 4.5 g **Sodium:** 410 mg (without salt)
(3 PointsPlus | 3 SmartPoints | 0 SmartPoints on FreeStyle Plan or FlexPlan)

0FS - Turkey Pumpkin Chili

(Prep time:20 min | Cook time:1 h | Total time:1 h20 min | Serves: 8)
INGREDIENTS:
- 1 pound 99% lean ground turkey
- 3/4 cup chopped onions
- 1/2 cup chopped green bell peppers
- 2 cloves garlic, minced
- 2 (14.5 ounce) cans diced tomatoes, with liquid
- 1 (15 ounce) can unsweetened pure pumpkin puree
- 1 (15 ounce) can kidney beans, with liquid
- 1 (15 ounce) can Great Northern beans, with liquid
- 1 (15 ounce) can tomato sauce
- 1 (4 ounce) can diced green chiles
- 2 teaspoons ground chili powder
- 1 1/2 teaspoons ground cumin (or more to taste)
- 1 teaspoon salt
- 1/2 teaspoon ground black pepper
- 1 1/2 teaspoons oregano
- 1/2 cup water

DIRECTIONS:
1. Brown meat in large pot. Remove meat and place on paper towels to remove excess fat. Wipe any remaining fat from the pot and coat pot with cooking spray.
2. Sauté onion, bell pepper and garlic; sauté until tender. Return meat to pot. Add all remaining ingredients and stir to combine. Simmer 30 minutes to 1 hour. If chili is too thick for you, add more water, and adjust seasonings as needed.

Nutritional Information per serving (Serving size: Recipe divided into 8 equal portions) Calories: 276, Fat: 6g, Saturated Fat: 1.5g, Sugar: 4g, Fiber: 5.25g, Protein: 20g, Carbohydrates: 39g
0 SmartPoints on FreeStyle Plan

0FS - Slow Cooker Black Beans

(Prep time: 5 min | Cook time: 8 h | Total time: 8 h 5 min | Serves: 10)

Ingredients
- 2 cups dry black beans
- 1 onion, quartered
- 4 garlic cloves, peeled
- 2 jalapeno peppers, whole
- 1 bay leaf
- 1 tsp. salt

Nutritional Facts
Serving Size:
1/2 cup
Amount Per Serving
Calories 140, Total Fat 1g, Saturated Fat 0g, Total Carbohydrate 26g Dietary Fiber 6g, Sugars 1g, Protein 9g

Directions
1. Add everything to the slow cooker. Cover the beans with water or stock until there is one inch of water over the beans.
2. Cook on low for 8 hours.

0 SmartPoints on FreeStyle Plan or FlexPlan

0FS - Crock Pot Chicken Taco Chili

(Prep time: 10 min | Cook time: 10 min | Total time: 6 h | Serves: 5)
INGREDIENTS:

- 1 small onion, chopped
- 1 (15.5 oz.) can black beans, drained
- 1 (15.5 oz.) can kidney beans, drained
- 1 (8 oz.) can tomato sauce
- 10 oz. package frozen corn kernels
- 2 (10 oz.) cans diced tomatoes w/chilies
- 4 oz. can chopped green chili peppers, chopped
- 1 packet reduced sodium taco seasoning or homemade (see below)
- 1 tbsp. cumin
- 1 tbsp. chili powder
- 24 oz. (3) boneless skinless chicken breasts
- 1/4 cup chopped fresh cilantro

To make your own taco seasoning, omit the packet, cumin and chili powder above and use below instead:
- 1 1/2 tablespoons cumin
- 1 1/2 tablespoons chili powder
- 1/4 teaspoon garlic powder
- 1/4 teaspoon onion powder
- 1/4 teaspoon dried oregano
- 1/2 teaspoon paprika
- 1 teaspoon kosher salt
- 1/2 teaspoon black pepper

DIRECTIONS:
1. Combine beans, onion, chili peppers, corn, tomato sauce, diced tomato, cumin, chili powder and taco seasoning in a slow cooker and mix well.
2. Nestle the chicken in to completely cover and cook on LOW for 8 to 10 hours or on HIGH for 4 to 6 hours.
3. Half hour before serving, remove chicken and shred.
4. Return chicken to slow cooker and stir in.
5. Top with fresh cilantro and your favorite toppings!

NUTRITION INFORMATION
Yield: 10 servings, Serving Size: About 1 cup
- **Amount Per Serving:**

Calories: 220, Total Fat: 3g, Saturated Fat: g
Carbohydrates: 28g, Fiber: 8.5g, Sugar: 6g, Protein: 21g
0 SmartPoints on FreeStyle Plan

0FS - Authentic Shoyu Ahi Poke

(Prep time:5 min | Cook time:0 min | Total time:5 min | Serves: 5)
TOTAL TIME: 5 minutes

Shoyu Ahi Poke is the traditional Hawaiian dish of raw fish seasoned with soy sauce and sesame oil.

INGREDIENTS:
- 1 lbs. sushi grade tuna, cut into 3/4 inch cubes
- 1/4 cup thin sliced onions
- 1/2 cup sliced scallions, green parts only
- 2 tbsp. reduced sodium soy sauce* (use coconut aminos for Whole30/Paleo)
- 1 teaspoon sesame oil
- 1/2 teaspoon sambal oelek or sriracha

DIRECTIONS:
1. In a medium bowl combine all the ingredients and gently fold until mixed well.
2. Serve immediately or cover tight and refrigerate for up to a day.
3. If you let it marinate, you may need to add another splash of soy sauce to taste.

*use gluten-free soy sauce for gluten-free diets.

NUTRITION INFORMATION
Yield: 4 servings, Serving Size: 1/4 lbs. poke only (veggies extra)
- **Amount Per Serving:**

Calories: 166, Total Fat: 4g, Saturated Fat: g, Carbohydrates: 2.5g Fiber: 0.5g, Sugar: 0.6g, Protein: 28.5g

0 SmartPoints on FreeStyle Plan

0FS - Red Pepper Muffin Tin Eggs

(Prep time:10 min | Cook time:40 min | Total time:50 min | Serves: 12)

Ingredients
- 12 eggs
- 1 teaspoon Montreal Steak Seasoning Blend
- 1 red, orange, or green pepper, diced
- ½ pound 99% fat-free ground turkey breast
- ½ teaspoon sage
- ½ teaspoon salt

- ½ teaspoon black pepper
- ¼ teaspoon red pepper flakes
- ¼ teaspoon marjoram
- Non-Stick Cooking Spray

Instructions

1. Preheat oven to 350 degrees.
2. Spray a muffin tin with non-stick spray.
3. Spray a large non-stick skillet with non-stick spray. On medium heat cook ground turkey, sage, salt, black pepper, red pepper flakes, and marjoram for 7-10 minutes or until cooked through. Stir consistently to prevent sticking.
4. While turkey is cooking, in a large bowl, beat eggs and Montreal steak seasoning together until well mixed and fluffy (2-3 minutes). Stir in diced bell pepper.
5. Once the turkey is cooked through, spoon into the muffin tins spreading equally between each muffin tin.
6. Pour egg mixture over the turkey filling ¾ of the way full.
7. Bake at 350 degrees for 30 minutes.

Makes 6 Servings (2 muffin tin eggs per serving)

0 SmartPoints on FreeStyle Plan

0FS - Slow Cooked Chicken Verde

INGREDIENTS
1 Pound Boneless Skinless Chicken Breasts
6 Tomatillos peeled and quartered
2 Jalapenos Seeded
1/2 White Onion quartered
2 Tablespoons Minced Garlic
1/2 Cup Fat-Free Low Sodium Chicken Broth
1 Tablespoon Cumin
1 Teaspoon Salt
1 Teaspoon Black Pepper

DIRECTIONS
In blender purée all ingredients except for chicken until a slightly chunky.
- Place chicken in bottom of crock pot and pour purée over top
- Cook on low heat for 6 hours
- Shred chicken and serve with extra sauce over top

Makes 6 servings
0 SmartPoints on FreeStyle Plan

0FS - Crockpot Tomato Balsamic Chicken

(Prep time:10 min | Cook time:4 h | Total time:4 h, 10 min | Serves: 6)

Ingredients
- 2 lbs. boneless and skinless chicken breast
- 28 oz. canned diced tomatoes, half of liquid drained
- 1 sweet onion, sliced thin
- 4 garlic cloves, minced
- 3 tbsp. balsamic vinegar (plus more for serving)
- 1 tbsp. Italian seasoning
- 6 cups fresh spinach
- Salt and pepper

Nutritional Facts
Serving Size:
3/4 cup
Amount Per Serving
Calories 227

Calories from Fat 14
Total Fat 2g
Saturated Fat 0g
Total Carbohydrate 12g
Dietary Fiber 3g
Sugars 7g
Protein 35g
Directions
1. Add the chicken to the slow cooker. Season with salt and pepper. Stir in the remaining ingredients except the spinach.
2. Cook on low for 4 hours adding the spinach during the last 30 minutes of cooking.

0 SmartPoints on FreeStyle Plan or FlexPlan

0FS - Slow Cook Chicken Cacciatore

INGREDIENTS:
- 8 bone-in, skinless chicken thighs
- 3/4 teaspoon kosher salt
- freshly ground black pepper
- cooking spray
- 5 garlic cloves, finely chopped
- 1/2 large onion, chopped
- 1 28-ounce can crushed tomatoes
- 1/2 medium red bell pepper, chopped
- 1/2 medium green bell pepper, chopped
- 4 ounce sliced shiitake mushrooms
- 1 sprig of fresh thyme
- 1 sprig of fresh oregano
- 1 bay leaf
- 1 tablespoon chopped fresh parsley (I omitted this)
- freshly grated Parmesan cheese, for serving (optional)

DIRECTIONS:
1. Season the chicken with salt and pepper to taste. Heat a large nonstick skillet over medium-high heat.
2. Coat with cooking spray, add the chicken, and cook until browned- 2 to 3 minutes per side. Transfer to your slow cooker.

3. Reduce the heat under the skillet to medium and coat with more cooking spray. Add the garlic and onion and cook, stirring, until soft- 3 to 4 minutes.
4. Transfer to the slow cooker and add the tomatoes, bell peppers, mushrooms, thyme, oregano and bay leaf. Stir to combine.
5. Cover and cook on high for 4 hours or on low for 8 hours.
6. Discard the bay leaf and transfer the chicken to a large plate. Pull the chicken meat from the bones (discard the bones), shred the meat, and return it to the sauce.
7. Stir in the parsley (if using). If desired, serve topped with Parmesan cheese.

Nutritional information per serving: Calories: 220, Fat: 6g, Sat Fat: 1.5g, Cholesterol: 123mg, Sodium: 319mg, Carbohydrates: 10g, Fiber: 2g, Sugar: 6g, Protein: 31g
Weight Watchers POINTS: Freestyle SmartPoints: 0 (but only if you use chicken breast instead of thighs)

0FS - Succotash Bean Soup

(Prep time:10 min | Cook time:10 min | Total time:20 min | Serves: 5)
(12 approximately 1 cup servings)
Ingredients:
2 cans white beans (rinsed and drained)
2 cans Lima beans (rinsed and drained)
2 cans corn kernels drained
1 carton low sodium vegetable broth
12 slices Canadian bacon chopped into small pieces
Season to taste

Instructions
Dump all ingredients into a large crockpot. Stir gently to evenly mix ingredients. Cook on low 6-8 hours. This is zero points...you have enough left for cornbread!
0 SmartPoints on FreeStyle Plan or FlexPlan

1FS - Healthy Tuna Salad Wraps

(Prep time:5 min | Cook time:5 min | Total time:10 min | Serves: 2)

Ingredients
- 1 12oz can Tuna, in water low sodium
- 1 egg, hard boiled
- ¼ Small Onion, chopped
- 1 Teaspoon Dill Pickle Relish
- 2 Tablespoons Greek Yogurt, Plain
- 1 Teaspoon Mayonnaise
- ½ Teaspoon Garlic Powder
- ½ Teaspoon Black Pepper
- ¼ Teaspoon Salt
- Fresh Bib Lettuce for "wraps"
- Tomatoes for garnish

Instructions
1. Drain water from tuna.
2. Pour drained tuna into a medium bowl and mix with all ingredients except tomato and lettuce.
3. Scoop into lettuce "wraps" and top with sliced tomatoes.

Makes 2 Servings
1 SmartPoints on FreeStyle Plan or FlexPlan

1FS - Cheesy Veggie Egg Scramble

(Prep time:5 min | Cook time:10 min | Total time:15 min | Serves: 6)

Ingredients
- 6 Large Eggs (Cage Free)
- 1 Organic Tomato Diced
- 3 Cups Organic Baby Spinach
- ½ Organic Red Onion Diced
- 1 Clove Garlic Crushed & Minced
- 1 Teaspoon Fresh Cracked Black Pepper
- 1 Teaspoon Kosher Salt
- ½ Cup Organic 2% Sharp Cheddar Cheese (we love Cabot brand)
- 1½ Tablespoons Organic Extra Virgin Olive Oil

Instructions
1. In a large bowl, beat together eggs, black pepper, and salt, set aside.
2. Bring olive oil to temperature in large skillet

3. Add in tomato, spinach, onion, and garlic and sauté for 5-7 minutes or until veggies are cooked through.
4. Pour beaten eggs over vegetables and cook for additional 3-4 minutes stirring occasionally. Cook until egg is set.
5. Remove from heat and sprinkle with cheese.

Makes 6 Servings
1 SmartPoints on FreeStyle Plan or FlexPlan

1FS - White Bean Turkey Chili

(Prep time:15 min | Cook time:60 min | Total time:75 min | Serves: 8)

Ingredients
- 2 cups shredded cooked turkey
- ½ cup diced onion
- ½ green pepper, diced
- ½ cup diced celery
- 2 tablespoons olive oil
- 1 tablespoon minced garlic
- 2 cups chicken broth
- 3 cans (15-16 oz.) white beans / great northern beans
- ¼ teaspoon cayenne pepper
- 1 teaspoon ground cumin
- ¾ teaspoon oregano
- ½ teaspoon salt
- ¼ teaspoon ground black pepper
- shredded Parmesan cheese, sour cream, and cilantro for serving if desired

Instructions
1. In a large stock pot or Dutch oven, add onion, green pepper, celery and olive oil. Cook on medium-high heat until onions are translucent and peppers are tender. Stir in garlic.
2. Add chicken broth, beans, and turkey and mix well. Stir in seasonings. Heat to boiling then reduce heat to simmer and cover for 30-60 minutes, stirring occasionally.
3. Heat to boiling then reduce heat to simmer and cover for 30-60 minutes, stirring occasionally.
4. Serve with sour cream, cheese, and cilantro.

Makes 8 Servings (approximately 1 cup each)

1 SmartPoints on FreeStyle Plan or FlexPlan

1FS - Sweet & Sour Meatballs

(Prep time:5 min | Cook time:15 min | Total time:20 min | Serves: 6)

Ingredients
- 1 pound 99% Ground Turkey breast or Ground Chicken Breast
- ½ Teaspoon Salt
- 1 Teaspoon Black Pepper
- 1 Teaspoon Onion Powder
- 1 Teaspoon Garlic Powder
- 1 Teaspoon Paprika
- 1 Teaspoon Cumin
- ¼ teriyaki sauce
- ¼ Cup Sugar-Free BBQ Sauce
- ⅛ cup apple cider vinegar
- 1 tablespoon brown sugar twin

Instructions
1. In a large bowl, mix together ground meat and spices (salt, pepper, onion powder, garlic powder, paprika, and cumin).Mix until well blended.
2. In a small bowl, mix together the teriyaki sauce, BBQ sauce, apple cider vinegar, and brown sugar twin.
3. Add ¼ cup of sauce mixture to meat mixture and mix well.
4. Roll meat mixture into 1½" balls.Should make about 12 meatballs
5. Place meatballs on a lined baking sheet (we use silicone baking mats) about 1" apart
6. Bake at 375 degrees for 10 minutes.Turn meatballs, and cook for additional 10 minutes.
7. Remove from oven and toss with sauce until well coated.

Makes 6 servings of 3 meatballs per serving
1 SmartPoints on FreeStyle Plan or FlexPlan

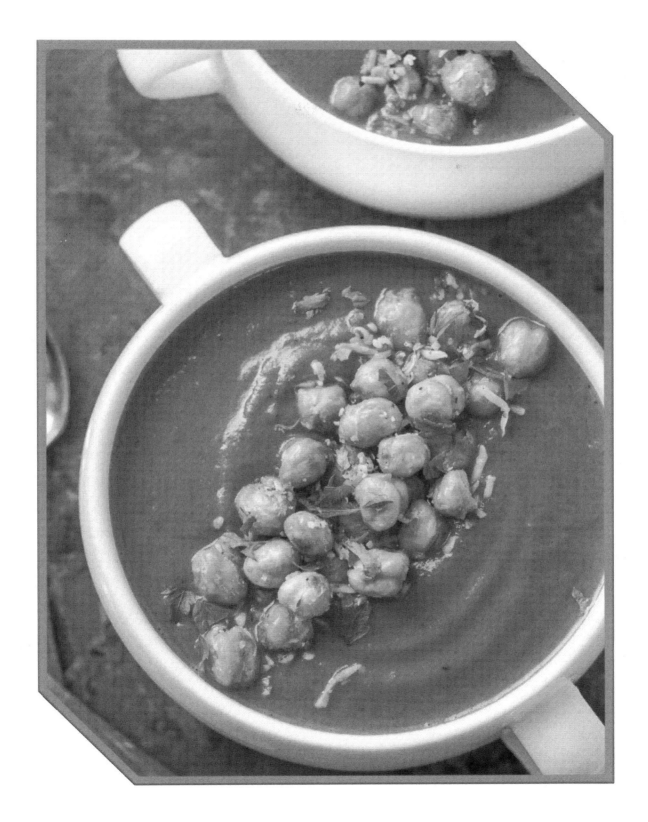

5FSP - Raspberry Chicken Salad

Serves: 4
5 SmartPoints™

Ingredients:
6 cup mixed greens (arugula, endive, spinach, etc.)
2 cups cooked chicken, shredded or cubed
¼ cup walnuts, chopped
1 cup fresh raspberries
½ cup feta cheese

Directions:
1. Thoroughly rinse the greens and combine them in a bowl. Toss to mix.
2. Add the chicken and walnuts to the bowl and toss again.
3. At this point, you can either keep all of the ingredients in the large bowl for serving or transfer the salad to individual serving plates.
4. Top the salad with fresh raspberries and crumbled feta cheese.
5. Serve immediately while the greens are still crisp.

Nutritional Information:
Calories 197, Total Fat 10.7 g, Saturated Fat 3.7 g, Total Carbohydrate 5.4 g, Dietary Fiber 4.1 g, Sugars 0.9 g, Protein 17.7 g

5FS - Asparagus and Chicken Salad

Serves: 4
5 SmartPoints™

Ingredients:
1 ½ pounds fresh asparagus, trimmed
12 endive leaves, trimmed
2 cups chicken, cooked and sliced
½ teaspoon salt, optional
½ teaspoon black pepper, optional
¼ cup stilton cheese crumbles
½ lemon, zested and juiced

Directions:
1. Place the asparagus spears in a skillet and add just enough water to cover.
2. Turn the heat on to medium-high and bring the water to a boil. Cover, reduce the heat to low and simmer for approximately 5 minutes, or until the asparagus is firm tender.
3. Remove the asparagus from the pan and immediately place it in a bowl of cold water for 1 minute.
4. Remove the asparagus from the water, drain well and set aside.
5. Arrange 3 endive leaves on each plate, topped with the sliced chicken.
6. Season with salt and pepper, if desired.
7. Next, sprinkle on the stilton cheese crumbles and top with the asparagus.
8. Drizzle with lemon juice to your liking and garnish with lemon zest before serving.

Nutritional Information:
Calories 181, Total Fat 7.0 g, Saturated Fat 4.0 g, Total Carbohydrate 10.4 g, Dietary Fiber 6.8 g, Sugars 0.3 g, Protein 21.0 g

4FS - Simple Taco Salad

Serves: 4
4 SmartPoints™

Ingredients:
½ pound ground beef
½ teaspoon salt
1 teaspoon black pepper
½ teaspoon garlic powder
1 teaspoon cumin
½ cup fresh corn kernels
1 cup tomatoes, cubed
1 avocado, cubed
5 cups lettuce or salad mix, chopped
Fresh lime quarters for garnish, optional

Directions:
1. Place the ground beef in a skillet over medium heat.
2. Cook until the meat is completely browned, approximately 7-10 minutes. Drain off any excess fat. Season the meat with salt, black pepper, garlic powder, and cumin.
3. In a bowl, combine the cooked ground beef, fresh corn kernels, tomatoes, avocado and chopped lettuce. Toss gently to mix.
4. Serve the salad with fresh lime wedges for dressing the salad, if desired.

Nutritional Information:
Calories 258, Total Fat 18.9 g, Saturated Fat 5.7 g, Total Carbohydrate 11.2 g, Dietary Fiber 5.1 g, Sugars 0.8 g, Protein 13.0 g

4FS - Chicken and Spinach Rings

Serves: 8
4 SmartPoints™
Ingredients:
5 ounces grilled chicken, cut in strips
1 cup baby spinach, fresh
1 (8 ounce) can crescent roll dough (reduced fat)
4 tablespoons whipped cream cheese (reduced fat), softened
⅓ Cup Mexican blend cheese (reduced fat), shredded
Spices of your choice

Directions:
1. Preheat the oven to 375°F.
2. Arrange the crescent roll dough, unrolled, on an ungreased baking sheet. Spread the cream cheese on each, and then season with your favorite spices.
3. Place the spinach on top of the cream cheese and lay on the grilled chicken strips. Sprinkle with the Mexican blend cheese. Make the rings by pulling the ends of each crescent roll up and wrapping it around the filling. Tuck them so they retain the shape.

4. Bake for 14 minutes, or until the crescent rolls become golden brown.

Nutritional Information:
Calories 142, Total Fat 5.0 g, Saturated Fat 2.0 g, Total Carbohydrate 16.0 g, Dietary Fiber 1.0 g, Sugars 1.0 g, Protein 8.0 g

5FS - Chicken Club Salad

Serves: 4
5 SmartPoints™

Ingredients:
8 cups mixed dark salad greens
1 pound chicken, cooked and sliced
½ cup bacon, cooked and diced
2 cups heirloom tomatoes, cut into wedges
½ cup fat free ranch dressing

Directions:
1. Place the salad greens in a bowl and add the fat free ranch dressing. Toss to coat.
2. Next, add the chicken, bacon, and tomatoes. Toss to mix.
3. Serve immediately, or cover and refrigerate for up to two hours before serving.

Nutritional Information:
Calories 215, Total Fat 4.6 g, Saturated Fat 1.3 g, Total Carbohydrate 11.0 g, Dietary Fiber 1.3 g, Sugars 5.2 g, Protein 28.1 g

6FS - Roasted Caprese Salad Chicken

Serves: 4
6 SmartPoints™

Ingredients:
4 cups heirloom grape tomatoes, halved
1 ½ tablespoons olive oil
1 teaspoon salt, divided
1 teaspoon black pepper, divided
1 pound boneless, skinless chicken breast, cooked and sliced

1 cup fresh mozzarella bocconcini
½ cup fresh basil, torn
1 tablespoon balsamic vinegar

Directions:

1. Preheat the oven to 400°F and line a baking sheet with parchment paper or aluminum foil.

2. Wash the grape tomatoes and cut each in half.

3. Drizzle the olive oil over the tomatoes and season with half a teaspoon each of salt and black pepper. Toss to mix.

4. Spread the tomatoes out on the baking sheet and place in the oven. Cook for 10-12 minutes. Remove from the oven and allow to cool slightly.

5. Place the tomatoes in a bowl and combine them with the chicken, fresh mozzarella, and basil. Drizzle the salad with the balsamic vinegar and season with the remaining salt and black pepper. Toss gently.

6. Serve immediately, or cover and refrigerate for 30 minutes before serving.

Nutritional Information:
Calories 276, Total Fat 14.1 g, Saturated Fat 5.5 g, Total Carbohydrate 3.5 g, Dietary Fiber 0.0 g, Sugars 1.5 g, Protein 30.7 g

5FS - Fresh Egg Salad

Serves: 4
5 SmartPoints™

Ingredients:
4 large eggs
2 large egg whites
2 tablespoon mayonnaise (reduced-calorie)
1 teaspoon fresh dill, shopped
2 tablespoon fresh chives, chopped
½ teaspoon Dijon mustard
½ teaspoon table salt or to taste
¼ teaspoon black pepper, freshly ground

Directions:

1. Place all 6 eggs in a saucepan and add water to cover.

2. Cover the saucepan with a lid and set it over high heat to boil. Boil for about 10 minutes, and drain the water. Place the eggs in ice water to cool so you'll be able to handle them. When the eggs are cool, remove and discard the shells from all the 6 eggs and the yolks of 2 eggs, keeping the egg whites.

3. Cut the 4 whole eggs and the 2 egg whites into ½-inch pieces with a knife or an egg slicer. Transfer the cut eggs to a medium bowl and add the mayonnaise, dill, chives, mustard, salt and pepper. Mix all the ingredients together until they have blended well. Serve and enjoy.

Nutritional Information:
Calories 106, Total Fat 7.3 g, Saturated Fat 1.9 g, Total Carbohydrate 1.3 g, Dietary Fiber 0.1 g, Sugars 1.0 g, Protein 8.2 g

4FS - Fruit & Blue Cheese Tossed Salad

Serves: 4
4 SmartPoints™

Ingredients:
4 tablespoons balsamic vinegar
4 teaspoons maple syrup
Salt to taste
2 tablespoons olive oil
6 cups mixed baby spinach leaves
2 medium pears, sliced
¼ cup blue cheese, chopped
1 tablespoon pine nuts (optional)

Directions:
1. Mix the vinegar, maple syrup, salt, and olive oil in a small bowl. Mix well until everything has combined properly.

2. Mix the baby spinach, lettuce, and pears in a large bowl and sprinkle the salad with the dressing. Toss to coat.

3. Spread the blue cheese and the pine nuts on top of the salad. Serve immediately.

Nutritional Information:
Calories 149, Total Fat 9.7 g, Saturated Fat 2.6 g, Total Carbohydrate 15.0 g, Dietary Fiber 3.6 g, Sugars 7.0 g, Protein 3.4 g

7FS - Sweet Potato Chili

Serves: 4
7 SmartPoints™

Ingredients:
2 teaspoons olive oil
1 cup red onion, diced
4 cups sweet potatoes, peeled and cut into small cubes
1 teaspoon salt
1 teaspoon coarse ground black pepper
1 tablespoon chili powder
½ teaspoon cinnamon
2 cups black beans, cooked or canned
4 cups vegetable stock
2 cups fresh or jarred salsa
Fresh cilantro for garnish (optional)

Directions:
1. Place the olive oil in a large saucepan or stock pot over medium heat.
2. Add the onions and sauté for 3 minutes.
3. Add the sweet potatoes, salt, black pepper, chili powder and cinnamon. Cook, stirring frequently, for 3 minutes.
4. Next add the remaining ingredients including the black beans, vegetable stock, and salsa. Mix well.
5. Increase the heat to medium high and cook until the liquid begins to boil. Cover and reduce the heat to low. Simmer for 20 minutes, or until the sweet potatoes are tender.
6. Serve warm, garnished with fresh cilantro, if desired.

Nutritional Information:
Calories 324, Total Fat 3.7 g, Saturated Fat 0.6 g, Total Carbohydrate 71.1 g, Dietary Fiber 16.3 g, Sugars 2.5 g, Protein 15.7 g

6FS - Roasted Cauliflower Soup

Serves: 6, 6 SmartPoints™

Ingredients:
8 cups cauliflower florets (approximately one large head)
1 cup yellow onion, sliced
1 cup fennel bulb, sliced
2 tablespoons olive oil
2 teaspoons fresh rosemary, chopped
½ teaspoon nutmeg
1 teaspoon salt
1 teaspoon black pepper
6 cups vegetable stock
½ cup pancetta, diced

Directions:

1. Preheat the oven to 450°F and line a baking sheet with aluminum foil.

2. In a bowl, toss together the cauliflower, onion, and fennel. Drizzle the vegetables with olive oil and season with rosemary, nutmeg, salt, and black pepper. Toss to mix.

3. Spread the vegetables out on a baking sheet and place them in the oven. Bake for 15 minutes.

4. While the vegetables are roasting, bring the vegetable stock to a boil in a soup pot over medium high heat.

5. Place the pancetta in a small skillet over medium heat, and cook for 3-5 minutes, stirring frequently, until lightly crispy.

6. Remove the vegetables from the oven and carefully transfer to the boiling vegetable stock. Cover, reduce the heat to low and simmer for 10-14 minutes.

7. Working in batches, transfer the soup to a blender or food processor and puree before adding the soup back to the pot. Continue with the remaining soup until the desired consistency has been reached.

8. Serve warm, garnished with crispy pancetta.

Nutritional Information:
Calories 196, Total Fat 8.2 g, Saturated Fat 2.0 g, Total Carbohydrate 25.8 g, Dietary Fiber 9.4 g, Sugars 3.8 g, Protein 8.9 g

5FS - Mushroom Egg Drop Soup

Serves: 4
5 SmartPoints™
Ingredients: 4 cups chicken stock
5 wonton wrappers
1 cup oyster mushrooms, thinly sliced
2 eggs, beaten
1 teaspoon soy sauce
½ teaspoon salt
1 teaspoon white pepper
Scallions, sliced for garnish (optional)
Lime slices for garnish (optional)Directions:

1. Place the chicken stock in a soup pan and bring it to a boil over medium-high heat. Once the stock comes to a boil, reduce the heat to medium low.

2. While the stock is coming to a boil, lay the wonton wrappers out on the counter and slice them into ½-inch thick pieces.

3. Add the mushrooms and sliced wonton wrappers to the chicken stock and cook for 1-2 minutes.

4. In a bowl, combine the beaten eggs, soy sauce, salt, and white pepper. Whisk together.

5. Slowly pour the egg mixture into the soup, whisking constantly to create thin strips of cooked egg throughout the soup. Cook for an additional 1-2 minutes.

6. Remove the soup from the heat and serve warm, garnished with scallions and lime, if desired.

Nutritional Information:
Calories 151, Total Fat 5.3 g, Saturated Fat 1.6 g, Total Carbohydrate 15.1 g, Dietary Fiber 0.5 g, Sugars 3.9 g, Protein 10.4 g a

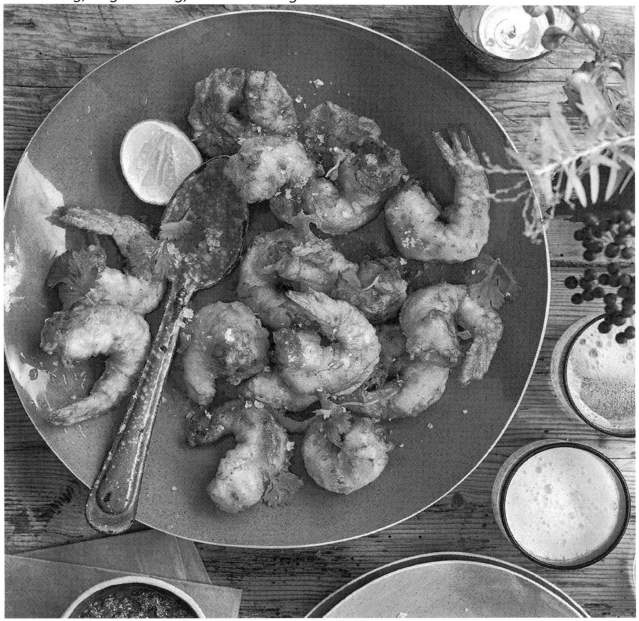

5FS - Tasty Turkey Meatball & Veggie

Makes 8 servings.
One serving is 1-1/2 cups soup.
One serving is 5 FreeStyle WW SP.
5 WW FreeStyle SP per serving.

INGREDIENTS
- Cooking spray
- 1 onion, chopped
- 3-4 carrots, sliced or chopped
- 1 cup green beans, cut
- 2 minced garlic cloves
- 1 (24 ounce) package Jennie-O Italian style turkey meatballs
- 2 (14.5 ounce) cans beef or vegetable broth
- 2 (14.5 ounce) diced or Italian stewed tomatoes
- 1-1/2 cups frozen corn
- 1 teaspoon oregano
- 1 teaspoon parsley
- ½ teaspoon basil

INSTRUCTIONS
1. Spray large saucepan or instant pot with cooking spray.
2. Add onions, carrots, green beans and garlic and cook over medium heat 2-3 minutes.
3. Mix in remaining ingredients.
4. If cooking on a stovetop, cover and cook over medium-low heat for 20 minutes, or until meatballs are heated through.
5. -OR-
6. If using an instant pot, press the "soup" button and cook on high pressure for 15 minutes. Vent to release pressure once cooked.
7. -OR-
8. Cook in a slow cooker for 5-6 hours on LOW.
9. Serve warm.
10. Refrigerate or freeze leftovers.

Nutrition Information
- Serves: 8 servings
- Serving size: 1-1/2 cup soup

Calories: 285, Fat: 13 g, Saturated fat: 4 g, Carbohydrates: 21 g
Sugar: 9 g, Protein: 19 g

5FS - Creamy-Tomato-Basil-Soup

Serves: 4
Ingredients
- 1 cup low sodium chicken broth (or vegetable broth if you prefer)
- 1 14 oz. can tomato puree
- 1 cup skim milk
- 4-5 leaves fresh basil
- 3 tsp. olive oil
- 1 stalk celery
- ½ cup onions
- 1 Tbsp. cornstarch
- 1-2 cloves garlic, crushed.
- pepper to taste

Instructions
1. Rough chop onions and celery, transfer them to a food processor or chopper and puree until fine.
2. Heat olive oil in a large pan over medium heat.
3. Add onion and celery mix to pan and sauté until they begin to become translucent.
4. Reduce heat to low and stir in garlic, pepper, chicken stock, and tomato puree, and cornstarch-simmer on low for 5 minutes.
5. Whisk in tomato puree and milk, top with basil leaves, simmer for an additional 10 minutes.
6. Serve topped with a dollop of Greek yogurt or a fresh chopped basil.
7. This makes approximately 4 -1/2 cup servings

Makes 2 large servings
5 SmartPoints per serving on FreeStyle Plan, and Flex Plan

1FS - Chicken Taco Soup Recipe

Prep time: 5 mins
Cook time: 30 mins
Total time: 35 mins
Serves: 8

Ingredients
- 2 Cups Shredded or Cubed Chicken
- 1 onion, diced
- 1 bell pepper, diced

- 1 poblano pepper, diced
- 2 tomatoes, chopped
- 1 tablespoon garlic, minced
- 6 cups fat free chicken broth
- 1 cup tomato sauce
- 1½ cups kidney beans or pinto beans
- 2 tablespoons taco/fajita seasoning
- 1 tablespoon olive oil

Instructions
1. In a large stockpot, sauté the onion, bell pepper, poblano pepper, and tomato for 5 minutes stirring regularly. You want the vegetables to be tender.
2. Mix in chicken, broth, tomato sauce, garlic, pinto beans, and seasonings.
3. Simmer on medium heat for 30 minutes, stirring occasionally.
4. Serve with preferred garnishes like cheese, sour cream, or tortilla chips.

WW Information:
Makes 8 Servings (approximately 2 cups each)
1 SmartPoint per serving on FreeStyle Plan or FlexPlan

5FS - Sticky Buffalo Chicken Tenders

Prep time: 10 mins, **Cook time:** 15 mins, **Total time:** 25 mins
Ingredients
- 1 pound boneless skinless chicken breasts, pounded to ½" thickness
- ¼ cup flour
- 3 eggs
- 1 cup Italian Seasoned Panko breadcrumbs
- ½ cup brown sugar
- ⅓ cup Frank's Red Hot Sauce
- ½ teaspoon Garlic Powder
- 3 tablespoons water

Instructions
1. Preheat oven to 425 degrees and spray a baking sheet with non-stick cooking spray or line with silicone baking mats.
2. Cut boneless skinless chicken breasts into strips or chunks (we find chunks hold coating better).

3. Add the chicken into a large Ziploc bag that contains just the flour. Shake to coat.
4. Place Panko breadcrumbs into a shallow bowl. In another shallow bowl, whisk eggs until combined well.
5. Dip flour coated chicken into eggs, then into Panko breadcrumbs to coat.
6. Place coated chicken on the prepared baking sheet. Spray tops with non-stick cooking spray.
7. Bake for 15 minutes for nuggets or 20 minutes for strips or until chicken is browned and cooked through.
8. While chicken is in the oven, you will make your sauce mixture.
9. In a medium saucepan, bring the brown sugar, garlic powder, water and Frank's red hot sauce to a boil. Remove from heat and stir well.
10. When chicken is cooked through, remove from the oven and toss with sauce. This will just coat the chicken.

Makes 6 Servings
5 SmartPoints per Serving on FreeStyle or Flex Plan

5FS - Garlic Roasted Garbanzo Beans

Prep time: 5 mins, Cook time: 45 mins, Total time: 50 mins
Ingredients
- 1 can garbanzo beans (chickpeas)
- 1 tablespoon olive oil
- 1 teaspoon salt
- 1 teaspoon garlic powder
- ½ teaspoon paprika

Instructions
1. Preheat oven to 375° Fahrenheit.
2. Line a baking sheet with a silicone baking mat or parchment paper.
3. Drain and rinse the garbanzo beans.
4. Pat garbanzo beans dry, pour into a large bowl.
5. Toss with olive oil, salt, garlic powder, and paprika until all are well coated.
6. Spread evenly over baking sheet.
7. Bake at 375° for 20 minutes. Turn chickpeas so they are evenly roasted (use a spatula to flip them or simply stir around but make sure they are in an even layer).
8. Place back in the oven at 375° for additional 25 minutes.

9. Allow the roasted garbanzo beans to cool before storing in an airtight container for snacking.

Makes approximately 3 servings
5 SmartPoints per 1/2 cup on FreeStyle, and Flex Plan

1FS - Sweet & Sour Turkey Meatballs

Prep time: 5 mins
Cook time: 15 mins
Total time: 20 mins
Serves: 6

Ingredients
- 1 pound 99% Ground Turkey breast or Ground Chicken Breast
- ½ Teaspoon Salt
- 1 Teaspoon Black Pepper
- 1 Teaspoon Onion Powder
- 1 Teaspoon Garlic Powder
- 1 Teaspoon Paprika
- 1 Teaspoon Cumin
- ¼ teriyaki sauce
- ¼ Cup Sugar-Free BBQ Sauce
- ⅛ cup apple cider vinegar
- 1 tablespoon brown sugar twin

Instructions
1. In a large bowl, mix together ground meat and spices (salt, pepper, onion powder, garlic powder, paprika, and cumin). Mix until well blended.
2. In a small bowl, mix together the teriyaki sauce, BBQ sauce, apple cider vinegar, and brown sugar twin.
3. Add ¼ cup of sauce mixture to meat mixture and mix well.
4. Roll meat mixture into 1½" balls. Should make about 12 meatballs
5. Place meatballs on a lined baking sheet (we use silicone baking mats) about 1" apart
6. Bake at 375 degrees for 10 minutes. Turn meatballs, and cook for additional 10 minutes.
7. Remove from oven and toss with sauce until well coated.

WW Information:
Makes 6 servings of 3 meatballs per serving
1 SmartPoint on FreeStyle Plan or Flex Plan

5FS - Roasted Sweet Potato Side Dish

Prep time: 5 mins, Cook time: 25 mins, Total time: 30 mins

Ingredients
- 2 Medium Sweet Potatoes
- ½ teaspoon salt
- Non-Stick Cooking Spray

Instructions
1. Preheat oven to 400 degrees.
2. Line baking sheet with silicone baking mat or spray with non-stick spray.
3. Clean sweet potatoes, and peel if desired. We usually leave the skin intact. Remove any blemishes or eyes if needed.
4. Slice sweet potatoes into ¼" thick medallions
5. Place sweet potatoes in a single layer on prepared baking sheet.
6. Sprinkle the tops lightly with salt.
7. Bake at 400 degrees for 15 minutes. Turn sweet potato medallions over and bake additional 10 minutes.

This recipe makes 4 servings.
Each serving is approximately 1/2 sweet potato.
4 PointsPlus per serving
5 SmartPoints per serving on Beyond the Scale
5 SmartPoints per serving on FreeStyle Plan or Flex Plan

7FS - Apple Cheddar Turkey Wraps

Yield: 1 WRAP

INGREDIENTS:
- 1 Flatout Light Original Flatbread
- 1-2 leaves green leaf lettuce, torn
- 2 oz. thinly sliced deli turkey
- 1 oz. sliced 50% reduced fat sharp cheddar cheese
- 1 ½ teaspoons apple cider vinegar
- ½ teaspoon canola oil
- ½ teaspoon honey
- A pinch of salt and pepper
- ¼ cup matchstick-sliced apple pieces (slice apple into thin, short sticks)
- 1/3 cup coleslaw mix (just the shredded veggies, undressed)

DIRECTIONS:

1. Lay the Flatout flatbread on a clean, dry surface and lay the torn lettuce down the center of the flatbread going the long way (starting at the rounded end and spreading down the length of the flatbread to the other rounded end). You can leave a bit of space at each end as you'll be folding them over, and you do not need to cover the whole flatbread, just an area down the middle. Top the lettuce with the sliced deli turkey and the cheddar cheese. *Make sure to leave an inch or so of room at each end.*
2. In a small mixing bowl, combine the vinegar, oil, honey, salt and pepper and stir until well combined. Add the apples and coleslaw and stir to coat. Lay the apple/coleslaw mixture on top of the other ingredients layered on the wrap.
3. Fold in the rounded ends of the flatbread over the filling. Then fold one of the long edges over the filling and continue to roll until the wrap is completely rolled up. Cut in half and serve.

WEIGHT WATCHERS FREESTYLE SMARTPOINTS:
7 per wrap (SP *calculated using the recipe builder on weightwatchers.com*)

NUTRITION INFORMATION:
277 calories, 26 g carbs, 8 g sugars, 9 g fat, 3 g saturated fat, 28 g protein, 10 g fiber

2FS - Tasty BBQ Apricot Chicken

Prep time: 5 mins, Cook time: 30 mins, Total time: 35 mins
Serves: 6

Ingredients
- 1 pound boneless skinless chicken breasts
- ½ cup sugar-free apricot jam
- ½ cup G Hughes Sugar Free BBQ Sauce
- 2 tablespoons low sodium soy sauce
- 1 teaspoon garlic powder
- 1 teaspoon onion powder
- 1 teaspoon ground ginger

Instructions
1. In a medium bowl, whisk together the jam, bbq sauce, soy sauce, and seasonings.
2. Line baking sheet with foil and place chicken breasts in even layer
3. Pour barbecue sauce over chicken making sure well covered.
4. Bake at 350 degrees for 30 minutes.

5. Remove from oven, and serve with favorite sides.

WW Information:
Makes 6 Servings (approximately 3oz each)
2 SmartPoints per serving on Freestyle or FlexPlan

7FS - Pizza Lasagna Roll-Ups

Yield: 8 PIECES

INGREDIENTS:
- 8 uncooked lasagna noodles
- 15 oz. can tomato sauce
- 1 cup pizza sauce
- ½ teaspoon Italian seasoning
- 1 lb. uncooked hot Italian poultry sausage, casings removed if present (I used Wegmans patties, you can use chicken or turkey sausage)
- 2 oz. turkey pepperoni, chopped (reserve 8 slices un-chopped for topping)
- 1 (15 oz.) container fat free Ricotta cheese
- 1 (10 oz.) package frozen chopped spinach, thawed and squeezed until dry
- 1 large egg
- 2 oz. 2% shredded Mozzarella cheese

DIRECTIONS:
1. Pre-heat the oven to 350. Lightly mist a 9×13 baking dish with cooking spray and set aside.
2. Boil and salt a large pot of water and cook lasagna noodles according to package instructions. Drain and rinse with cold water. Lay noodles flat on a clean dry surface and set aside.
3. In a mixing bowl, combine the tomato sauce, pizza sauce and Italian seasoning and stir together. Set aside.
4. Place the sausage in a large skillet over medium heat and cook until browned, breaking the meat up into small pieces as it cooks. When the sausage is cooked through, add the chopped pepperoni and 1/3 cup of the tomato sauce mixture and stir to combine. Remove from heat.

5. In a mixing bowl, combine the ricotta cheese, spinach and egg and stir until well combined. Spoon 1/3 cup of the cheese mixture onto each lasagna noodle and spread across the surface leaving a little room (about ½") at the far end with no toppings. Top the cheese layer on each noodle with the meat mixture from step four, evenly dividing the meat between the noodles. Starting with one end (not the one with space at the end), roll the noodle over the filling until it becomes a complete roll. Repeat with all noodles.
6. Spoon ½ cup of the tomato sauce mixture into the prepared baking dish and spread across the bottom. Place the lasagna rolls seam down in the dish and spoon or pour the remaining sauce over top. Sprinkle the Mozzarella over the top of the rolls and place a pepperoni on each one. Cover the dish with aluminum foil and bake for 40 minutes.

WEIGHT WATCHERS FREESTYLE SMARTPOINTS:
7 per serving (*SP calculated using the recipe builder on weightwatchers.com*)
NUTRITION INFORMATION:
289 calories, 31 g carbs, 9 g sugars, 8 g fat, 2 g saturated fat, 24 g protein, 4 g fiber

3FS - Savory Chicken Dump Soup

3 FreeStyle Smart Points per serving (approximately 12 servings / 1 cup each)

Ingredients:
- 1 pound (approx. 3-4) raw skinless boneless chicken thighs
- 1 pkg Trader Joe's frozen Multigrain Blend with Vegetables (if you don't have a TJ's first of all bless your heart.
- Second find another frozen mix with some similar combo to this: cooked grain barley, corn, spelt [wheat], whole rice ermes variety [red], whole rice ribe variety, whole rice-venus variety [black], salt), peas, carrots, water, zucchini, vinegar, extra virgin olive oil, onion, sugar, salt, pepper and totaling no more than 17 SP for the entire bag
- 2 cups (one small package) shredded cabbage
- 1 cup (one small carton fresh or one can) sliced mushrooms any type
- 6 cups water
- 2 tsp dry Italian seasoning

Directions

1. This first part I prep ahead and have on hand in the freezer for easy dumping. If you are anxious to try this right away though there is no need to wait! Just plan a little extra time so your family and friends don't pass out smelling all that yumminess while they stalk you in the kitchen with empty bowls in hand.
2. Add all of the chicken and 1/2 the water to a tall stock pot.
3. Bring everything to a boil for 10 minutes. Reduce to a heavy simmer (not boiling, but bubbling vigorously) and cover loosely with aluminum foil. Let simmer for approximately an hour.
4. Remove one thigh and test with a meat thermometer. If the internal temp is not at least 150 (you want 165 when everything is done!) return and continue simmering for 15 minute intervals until chicken is completely done. If you are making this for prep, remove from heat and allow to cool.
5. Pull chicken apart with two forks to shred or use a hand mixer to "shred" (I haven't used the hand mixer method but I want to try it!).
6. Return to the broth you have just made and then transfer all to a freezer safe container. If you are using immediately return everything to the stock pot and go to the next step.
7. With your stock and shredded chicken in the stock pot, next dump all of the remaining ingredients and stir.
8. Bring back up to a low boil for 10 minutes, then reduce heat and simmer for 30-45 minutes

5FS - Chicken Marsala MeatBall

5 Free Style Smart Points 248 calories
TOTAL TIME: 30 minutes
INGREDIENTS:
- 8 ounces sliced cremini mushrooms, divided
- 1 pound 93% lean ground chicken
- 1/3 cup whole wheat seasoned or gluten-free bread crumbs
- 1/4 cup grated Pecorino cheese
- 1 large egg, beaten
- 3 garlic cloves, minced
- 2 tablespoons chopped fresh parsley, plus more for garnish
- 1 teaspoon Kosher salt
- Freshly ground black pepper
- 1/2 tablespoon all-purpose flour

- 1/2 tablespoon unsalted butter
- 1/4 cup finely chopped shallots
- 3 ounces sliced shiitake mushrooms
- 1/3 cup Marsala wine
- 3/4 cup reduced sodium chicken broth

DIRECTIONS:
1. Preheat the oven to 400F.
2. Finely chop half of the Cremini mushrooms and transfer to a medium bowl with the ground chicken, breadcrumbs, Pecorino, egg, 1 clove of the minced garlic, parsley, 1 teaspoon kosher salt and black pepper, to taste.
3. Gently shape into 25 small meatballs, bake 15 to 18 minutes, until golden.
4. In a small bowl whisk the flour with the Marsala wine and broth.
5. Heat a large skillet on medium heat.
6. Add the butter, garlic and shallots and cook until soft and golden, about 2 minutes.
7. Add the mushrooms, season with 1/8 teaspoon salt and a pinch of black pepper, and cook, stirring occasionally, until golden, about 5 minutes.
8. Return the meatballs to the pot, pour the Marsala wine mixture over the meatballs, cover and cook 10 minutes.
9. Garnish with parsley.

NUTRITION INFORMATION
Yield: 5 servings, Serving Size: 5 meatballs with mushrooms
- Amount Per Serving:

Smart Points: 5, Calories: 248, Total Fat: 4g, Saturated Fat: 4g
Carbohydrates: 13g, Fiber: 1.5g, Sugar: 4.5g, Protein: 21g

4FS - Bruschetta Topped Balsamic Chicken

Yield: 4 SERVINGS
INGREDIENTS:
- 4 (6 oz.) raw boneless skinless chicken breasts or cutlets
- Salt and pepper, to taste

- ½ teaspoon dried oregano
- 2 teaspoons olive oil, divided
- ¾ cup balsamic vinegar
- 2 tablespoons sugar
- ¼ teaspoon salt
- 1 cup chopped cherry or grape tomatoes
- 1-2 tablespoons of sliced fresh basil
- 1 teaspoon minced garlic (or more to taste)

DIRECTIONS:
1. Pre-heat the oven to 400 degrees. Place the chicken breasts on a cutting board and if necessary, pound with a meat mallet to ensure an even thickness.
2. Sprinkle each breast with salt, pepper and oregano on each side.
3. Pour 1 ½ teaspoons of olive oil into a large skillet and bring over medium-high heat.
4. Place the breasts in the pan in a single layer and cook for 1-2 minutes on each side to lightly brown the outside of the chicken.
5. Mist a baking sheet with cooking spray and place the chicken breasts onto the sheet. Cover with aluminum foil and bake for 15 minutes.
6. While the chicken is baking, combine the balsamic vinegar, sugar and salt in a small saucepan and stir to combine. Bring to a boil over medium-high heat and then reduce the heat to medium low. Simmer for 10-15 minutes until the mixture has reduced and thickened and will coat the back of a spoon. Split the balsamic glaze into two small dishes.
7. When the chicken comes out of the oven, discard any extra liquid produced by the chicken. Use a pastry brush to brush the glaze from one of the dishes onto the chicken breasts. Place the baking sheet of chicken back in the oven, uncovered this time, for 5-10 minutes until the chicken is cooked through. Wash your pastry brush thoroughly.
8. Combine the chopped tomatoes, sliced basil, minced garlic and the remaining ½ teaspoon of olive oil in a bowl and add salt and pepper to taste. Stir to combine.
9. When the chicken breasts are done cooking, brush the second dish of balsamic glaze over the chicken breasts. Serve each breast topped with ¼ cup of the bruschetta tomato mixture.

WEIGHT WATCHERS FREESTYLE SMARTPOINTS:
4 per serving NUTRITION INFORMATION:
293 calories, 18 g carbs, 17 g sugars, 7 g fat, 1 g saturated fat, 39 g protein, 1 g fiber .

5FS - Ham & Apricot Dijon Glaze

5 Free Style Smart Points 145 calories
TOTAL TIME: 5 hours
INGREDIENTS:
- 1 (6 to 7 pound) Hickory smoked fully cooked spiral cut ham
- 5 tbsp. apricot preserves
- 2 tablespoons Dijon mustard

DIRECTIONS:
1. Make the glaze: Whisk 4 tablespoons of preserves and mustard together.
2. Place the ham in a 6-quart or larger slow cooker, making sure you can put the lid on. You may have to turn the ham on its side if your ham is too large.
3. Brush the glaze over the ham. Cover and cook on the LOW setting for 4 to 5 hours. Brush the remaining tablespoon of preserves over the ham the 30 minutes.

NUTRITION INFORMATION
Yield: 16, Serving Size: 3 ounces
- Amount Per Serving:

Smart Points: 5, Calories: 145, Total Fat: 7g, Saturated Fat: 1.5g
Carbohydrates: 12g, Fiber: 0g, Sugar: 11g, Protein: 15g

7 Day Meal Plan

Let's Start

Monday

Breakfast

- Half a pint of skimmed milk(284ml)-3 points
- Yogurt, oats and berries- virtually fat free plain yogurt(150g)-2 points, oats(15g)-1 point, and frozen or fresh berries-0 points

Lunch-chicken salad

- One medium(120g) grilled skinless chicken breast-4 points
- Mixed salad leaves-0 points
- Beetroot, cucumber, red onion and tomato- 0 points
- Two tbsp. of sweetcorn(60g)-2 points
- One tbsp. of sunflower oil(5 ml)- 1 point
- Apple- 0 points

Dinner

- 125g of extra lean minced pork, mixed with diced onion and red chili- 5 points
- A tsp(5ml) of sunflower oil-1 point
- Tinned tomatoes- 0 points
- Fresh coriander- 0 points
- A small portion(40g dry weight) of whole-wheat pasta- 4 points
- Drained fruit cocktail tinned in natural juice- 0 points
- 2 tbsp.(90g) of zero fat Greek yogurt- 1 point

Dessert

- Half a packet(6g) of sugar free jelly crystals- 0 points
- Pear- 0 points
- 125g of reduced fat cottage cheese- 2 points, with carrot sticks- 0 points

Tuesday

Breakfast

- Half a pint of skimmed milk(284ml)-3 points
- Peanut butter on toast- thick sliced whole meal bread, one slice(28g)- 2points, reduced fat peanut butter(15g)- 2 points, 200ml glass of orange juice- 2 points

Lunch- ham salad sandwich

- Two slices of Thick sliced whole meal bread(56g)- 4 points
- Two tsp of low fat spread(10g)- 1 point
- Three slices of pre-packed ham(33g)- 1 point

- A tsp(5g) of wholegrain mustard- 0 points
- Lettuce and tomato- 0 points
- Pear- 0 points

Dinner-Cod and feta ratatouille

- Ratatouille- garlic, onion, pepper and courgette roasted in a tsp of sunflower oil and mixed with tinned tomatoes- 1 point
- 125g of cod fillet- 2 points
- A medium portion(40g) of feta cheese- 3 points
- 150g of new potatoes, cooked- 3 points
- Orange- 0 points

*Put the cod fillet on top of the ratatouille in a small oven proof dish. Let it cook until the fish starts to flake, then crumble the feta on top and place back in the oven for a few more minutes.
You then serve with the new potatoes.

Dessert

- A 26g toffee bar- 2 points
- Banana- 0 points
- A mug of soup- 0 points

Wednesday

Breakfast

- Half a pint(284ml) of skimmed milk- 3 points
- 2 Weetabix(38g) with berries and banana- 3 points

Lunch- ham and pea omelet

- Two medium eggs(45g each)- 4 points
- Three slices(33g) of pre-packed ham- 1 point
- Onion and spinach- 0 points
- A tbsp.(35g) of peas- 1 point
- A tsp of sunflower oil- 1 point
- Lettuce and cherry tomatoes- 0 points
- Apple- 0 points

Dinner- salmon and new potatoes

- A medium salmon fillet(130g), baked, with sliced lemon- 6 points
- 200g new potatoes cooked and crushed with a tsp of sunflower oil and fresh drill- 5 points.
- Broccoli and leeks- 0 points
- Half a packet(6g) of sugar free jelly crystals- 0 points
- Drained fruit tinned in natural juice- 0 points

Dessert

- Grapes- 0 points
- Virtually fat free plain yogurt(150g)- 2 points
- Pear- 0 points

Thursday

Breakfast

- Half a pint of skimmed milk- 3 points
- Two Weetabix of 38g- 3 points
- Raisins(15g)- 1 point

Lunch- tuna salad

- Lettuce, cherry tomatoes- 0 points
- Blanched green beans- 0 points
- 150g of cooked new potatoes- 3 points
- An 80g can of drained egg, medium(45g), and a tsp boiled sunflower oil- 1 point
- Orange- 0 points

Dinner- ratatouille with couscous

- Ratatouille as made on day two- 2 points
- Whole-wheat couscous- a medium portion of 60g in dry weight- 6 points
- Spinach- 0 points
- Two tbsp.(70g) of chick peas- 2 points
- Fresh parsley- 0 points
- Drained and grilled pineapple juice tinned in natural juice- 0 points

*Prepare the couscous by seasoning with salt & pepper then mix in the chick peas, parsley & spinach. It is then served alongside the ratatouille.

Dessert

- Banana- 0 points
- A medium(125g) corn on the cob- 2 points
- Two tbsp. of 0% fat Greek yogurt(90g)- 1 point

Friday

Breakfast

- Half a pint of skimmed milk- 3 points
- Beans on toast- a slice of thick sliced whole meal bread(28g)- 2 points, two tsp(10g) of low fat spread- 1 point
- Three tbsp.(105g) of baked beans- 2 points
- Apple- 0 points

Lunch- soup and houmous

- Soup- 0 points
- Two tbsp.(60g) of reduced fat houmous- 4 points
- Cucumber and carrot sticks- 0 points
- 10 olives(30g)- 1 point
- Kiwi fruit- 0 points

Dinner- bacon and cheese omelet

- Two medium eggs of 45g each- 4 points
- Two bacon medallions(40g)- 1 point
- Onion- 0 points
- A 30g half fat cheddar cheese- 2 points
- A pot(65g) of low fat chocolate mousse- 2 points

Dessert

- A medium glass(175ml) of dry white wine spritzer with soda water- 4 points
- Banana- 0
- Pear-0

Saturday
Breakfast

- Half a pint of skimmed milk- 3 points
- Banana and honey yogurt- virtually fat free plain yogurt(150g)- 2 points
- Banana- 0 points
- A tsp(15g) of honey- 1 point

Lunch- tuna filled baked potato

- A 200g baked potato- 4 points
- An 80g can of drained tuna in brine or spring water- 1 point
- A tbsp. of reduced fat mayonnaise- 1 point
- Spring onion- 0 points
- A tbsp. of sweetcorn- 1 point
- Lettuce, cucumber, cherry tomatoes- 0 points
- Grapes- 0 points

Dinner-Quorn stir fry

- 2(102g) Quorn fillets- 2 points
- A medium portion(60g) of cooked egg noodles- 6 points
- Stir fry veggies- 0 points
- Two tbsp.(30ml) of soy sauce- 0 points
- Fresh fruit salad- 0 points

Dessert

- A pot(65g) of low fat chocolate mousse- 2 points
- A crumpet(60g), toasted and topped with 30g low fat soft cheese- 3 points
- Apple- 0 points

Sunday
Breakfast

- Half a pint of skimmed milk- 3 points

- Bacon, beans and egg- baked beans, three tbsp.(105g)-2 points, two(40g) bacon medallions- 1 point, a medium(45g) poached egg- 2 points
- A tbsp. of ketchup- 0 points

Lunch- cheese on toast

- A slice of whole meal bread(28g)- 2 points
- A 20g pickle- 1 point
- A 30g half fat cheddar cheese- 2 points
- Salad- 0 points
- Grapes- 0 points

Dinner- turkey steak with veggies and curry

- A medium(150g) turkey steak- 4 points
- Two tbsp. of prepared gravy granules- 1 point
- A 20g Yorkshire pudding- 1 point
- Cauliflower and carrots- 0 points
- Two tbsp. of peas- 2 points
- A small glass(125ml) of dry white wine with a dash of soda water- 3 points

Dessert

- 10 olives- 1 point
- Two tbsp. of 0% fat Greek yogurt with a sliced banana- 1 point
- Pear- 0 points

In the next section, I've included my favorite recipes that I could recommend, Although, points is of the old smart points system but never the less still usable and as tasty as always, so let enjoy!

WW Smart Points Main course Recipes

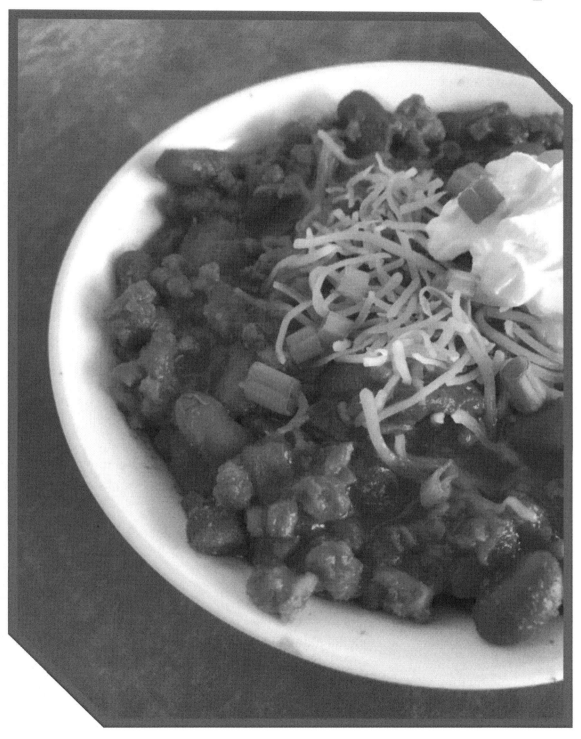

Honey Sesame Chicken

Serves: 4
6 SmartPoints™

Ingredients:
1 pound boneless, skinless chicken breast
2 teaspoons coconut oil
½ teaspoon salt
1 teaspoon coarse ground black pepper
½ teaspoon cayenne powder
1 tablespoon freshly grated ginger
2 tablespoons honey
¼ cup soy sauce
2 teaspoons sesame oil
1 tablespoon sesame seeds, toasted (optional)
Fresh lemongrass for garnish, optional
Cooked rice for serving (optional)

Directions:
1. Using a meat mallet, flatten the chicken until it is approximately ¼ inch thick.
2. Melt the coconut oil in a skillet over medium heat.
3. Season the chicken with salt, black pepper, and cayenne powder. Cook the chicken in the skillet for 4-5 minutes per side, or until it is no longer pink in the center.
4. In a small bowl, combine the fresh ginger, honey, soy sauce, and sesame oil. Mix well and pour the sauce over the chicken.

Chicken Fried Rice

Serves: 4
4 SmartPoints™

Ingredients:
4 large egg whites
12 ounces boneless, skinless chicken breast, cut in ½-inch pieces
½ cup carrot, diced
½ cup scallion (green and white parts), chopped

2 garlic cloves, minced
½ cup frozen green peas, thawed
2 cups cooked brown rice, hot
3 tablespoons soy sauce (low-sodium)

Directions:
1. Coat a large, nonstick skillet with cooking spray, and set it over medium-high heat.
2. Add the egg whites and stir frequently as you cook, until they are scrambled, about 3-5 minutes. Place the eggs on a plate and set them aside.
3. Remove the pan from the heat and coat it again with cooking spray and place it over medium-high heat.
4. Add the chicken and carrots and sauté for about 5 minutes or until the chicken is golden brown. Check that the chicken is cooked through before adding the other ingredients.
5. When the chicken is ready, add the chopped scallions, minced garlic, peas, cooked brown rice, the egg whites, and soy sauce. Stir until the ingredients have combined well and continue cooking until all the ingredients are well heated.
6. Serve and enjoy.

Nutritional Information:
Calories 178, Total Fat 2.0 g, Saturated Fat 0.8 g, Total Carbohydrate 21.0 g, Dietary Fiber 38.0 g, Sugars 2.0 g, Protein 18.0 g

Tasty Orange Chicken

Serves: 4
3 SmartPoints™

Ingredients:
2 teaspoons olive oil or cooking spray
¾ cup sweet yellow onion, sliced
1 cup red bell pepper, sliced
1 pound boneless, skinless chicken breast, cubed
½ teaspoon salt
1 teaspoon coarse ground black pepper
1 teaspoon garlic powder
¼ cup low sugar orange marmalade
2 tablespoons soy sauce
Cooked rice for serving (optional)

Directions:
1. Heat the olive oil or cooking spray in a skillet over medium heat.
2. Place the onion and red bell pepper in the skillet and cook for 3-5 minutes, or until the vegetables are just starting to become tender. Remove from the skillet and set aside.
3. Season the chicken with the salt, black pepper and garlic powder. Add the chicken to the skillet and cook, stirring occasionally, for 5-7 minutes.
4. While the chicken is cooking, combine the marmalade and soy sauce. Mix well and then add to the chicken. Toss to coat.
5. Add the vegetables back into the skillet and continue to cook for an additional 5-7 minutes, or until the chicken is cooked through.
6. Remove from the heat and serve warm with cooked rice, if desired.

Nutritional Information:
Calories 173, Total Fat 3.1 g, Saturated Fat 0.8 g, Total Carbohydrate 8.4 g, Dietary Fiber 0.9 g, Sugars 4.6 g, Protein 26.4 g

Chicken and Sweet Potato

Serves: 4
5 SmartPoints™

Ingredients:
2 teaspoons olive oil or cooking spray
4 cups sweet potatoes, peeled and shredded
1 cup sweet yellow onion, diced
1 cup red bell pepper, diced
1 teaspoon salt
1 teaspoon black pepper
1 teaspoon Cajun seasoning mix
2 cups boneless skinless chicken breast, cooked and shredded
2 cups tomatoes, chopped
Fresh scallions, sliced for garnish (optional)

Directions:
1. Heat the olive oil or cooking spray in a large skillet over medium-high heat.

2. In a bowl, combine the sweet potatoes, onion, and red bell pepper. Toss to mix.
3. Add the vegetable mixture to the skillet and cook for 5-7 minutes, stirring frequently.
4. Season the vegetables with salt, black pepper and Cajun seasoning. Using a spatula, press the vegetables firmly into the bottom of the pan. Reduce the heat to medium and let them cook, without disturbing them, for 5-7 minutes, or until a crust begins to form on the bottom of the vegetables.

Beef Soba Bowls

Serves: 4
8 SmartPoints™

Ingredients:
1 pound flank or skirt steak, thinly sliced
Cooking spray
1 teaspoon salt
1 teaspoon black pepper
1 teaspoon ground ginger
4 cups fresh snow peas, washed and trimmed
¼ cup soy sauce
1 cup beef stock
½ pound soba noodles, cooked
Fresh cilantro for garnish (optional)
Lime wedges for garnish (optional)

Directions:
1. Spray a large skillet with vegetable oil and heat over medium.
2. Add the steak slices and season with salt, black pepper, and ground ginger. Cook, stirring occasionally, for 5-7 minutes, or until the meat has reached the desired doneness.
3. Remove the steak from the pan and keep it warm.
4. Add the snow peas to the pan and sauté for 2-3 minutes.
5. Combine the beef stock and soy sauce and add them to the skillet. Cook for 2-3 minutes, or until the liquid comes to a low boil.
6. Add the cooked soba noodles and toss. Cook an additional 1-2 minutes, or until warmed through.
7. Transfer the noodles, broth, and snow peas to a serving bowl and top with slices of steak.
8. Garnish with fresh cilantro and lime wedges before serving, if desired.

Nutritional Information:
Calories 328, Total Fat 8.8 g, Saturated Fat 3.7 g, Total Carbohydrate 31.1 g, Dietary Fiber 2.1 g, Sugars 3.5 g, Protein 32.7 g

Baked Artichoke Chicken

Serves: 4
3 SmartPoints™

Ingredients:
1 pound chicken breast tenders
Cooking spray
1 teaspoon salt
1 teaspoon coarse ground black pepper
1 cup jarred artichoke hearts
1 cup heirloom tomatoes, chopped
3 cloves garlic, crushed and minced
½ cup fresh basil, torn
1 tablespoon olive oil

Directions:
1. Preheat the oven to 375°F and spray an 8x8 or larger baking dish.
2. Place the chicken tenders in an even layer in the baking dish and season with the salt and coarse ground black pepper.
3. Combine the artichoke hearts, tomatoes, garlic, and basil in a bowl. Drizzle in the olive oil and toss to mix.
4. Spread the artichoke mixture over the chicken.
5. Place in the oven and bake for 25-30 minutes, or until the chicken is cooked through.
6. Remove from the oven and let rest at least 5 minutes before serving.

Nutritional Information: *Calories 185, Total Fat 3.2 g, Saturated Fat 0.8 g, Total Carbohydrate 8.9 g, Dietary Fiber 2.0 g, Sugars 1.5 g, Protein 28.4 g*

Garlic Thai Chicken

Serves: 4
6 SmartPoints™

Ingredients:
1 pound chicken breast tenders
Cooking spray

¼ cup garlic chili sauce
2 tablespoons honey
1 teaspoon salt
1 teaspoon black pepper
2 cups asparagus spears, chopped
1 cup onion, sliced
1 tablespoon olive oil
Cooked rice for serving (optional)

Directions:
1. Preheat the oven to 375°F and spray an 8x8 or larger baking dish with cooking spray.
2. Place the chicken in a single layer in the baking dish and season with the salt and black pepper.
3. In a bowl, combine the garlic chili sauce and honey. Mix well.
4. Pour the sauce mixture over the chicken, using a basting brush to evenly distribute over each piece.
5. Add the asparagus and onion to the baking dish and drizzle with the olive oil.
6. Place the baking dish in the oven and bake for 25-30 minutes, or until the chicken is cooked through.
7. Remove from the oven and let rest for at least 5 minutes before serving.

Nutritional Information:
Calories 242, Total Fat 6.6 g, Saturated Fat 1.3 g, Total Carbohydrate 17.1 g, Dietary Fiber 2.6 g, Sugars 10.6 g, Protein 28.2 g

Pork Tenderloin with Broccoli

Serves 4
7 SmartPoints™

Ingredients
1 pork tenderloin, about 1 pound
Salt and freshly ground black pepper
2 bunches broccoli rabe (about 1 pound), trimmed
Cooking spray
2 tablespoons olive oil, divided
2 tablespoons balsamic vinegar

Directions

1. Preheat oven to the broil setting and set oven rack to the upper-middle position. Line a baking sheet with parchment paper and lightly spray with cooking spray.
2. Trim the pork tenderloin from all visible fat and cut into 8 even slices. Season with salt and pepper on both sides.
3. Place broccoli rabe on the baking sheet. Spray lightly with cooking spray. Place in the oven under the broiler for 6-10 minutes until tender and golden brown. Turn the broccoli rabe over halfway through the cooking, about 4-5 minutes.
4. Warm 1 tablespoon of olive oil in a large heavy bottomed sauté pan like a cast iron over medium-high heat. Fry the pork for 8-10 minutes, turning halfway or until cooked your preferred doneness. Take the pan off the heat and remove the pork to a serving plate. Cover lightly with foil to keep warm.
5. Deglaze the pan with the balsamic vinegar and remaining 1 tablespoon of olive oil. Whisk the bottom of the pan to release the browned bits of flavors into the sauce. Season to taste with salt and pepper.
6. To serve, place 2 slices of the pork tenderloin with a quarter of the broccoli rabe on a serving plate. Pour a quarter of the sauce over the meat and vegetables and serve.

Nutritional Information:
Calories 317, Total Fat 16.1 g, Saturated Fat 3.3 g, Total Carbohydrate 3.8 g, Dietary Fiber 2.8 g, Sugars 0 g, Protein 36.2 g

Easy Pork Piccata

Serves: 4
5 SmartPoints™
Ingredients:
1 pound pork medallions
1 tablespoon olive oil or cooking spray
½ teaspoon salt
1 teaspoon black pepper
2 cloves garlic, crushed and minced
2 tablespoon capers
¼ cup dry vermouth
¼ cup fresh lemon juice
1 tablespoon fresh chives for garnish (optional)
Directions:

1. Heat the olive oil or cooking spray in a skillet over medium heat.
2. Arrange the pork medallions in the skillet and season with salt and black pepper. Cook for 2-3 minutes per side, or until cooked through.
3. Remove the pork medallions from the heat and keep warm until ready to serve.
4. Add the garlic and capers to the skillet. Cook for 1 minute, stirring gently.
5. Add the vermouth and lemon juice. Continue to cook while stirring and scraping the pan for 1-2 minutes.
6. Remove the sauce from the heat and immediately pour it over the pork medallions for serving.
7. Serve garnished with fresh chives, if desired.

Nutritional Information: *Calories 252, Total Fat 9.4 g, Saturated Fat 2.4 g, Total Carbohydrate 0.2 g, Dietary Fiber 0.1 g, Sugars 0.0 g, Protein 33.4 g*

Tender Spiced Pulled Pork

Serves 6
5 SmartPoints™

Ingredients

<u>Rub</u>
1 tablespoon paprika
1-3 teaspoons ancho chili powder according to taste
1 teaspoon salt
1 teaspoon ground cumin
1 teaspoon dry oregano
½ teaspoon black pepper
¼ teaspoon cinnamon
¼ teaspoon dry coriander

<u>Other ingredients</u>
2 pounds pork tenderloin, trimmed
1 onion, diced
4 garlic cloves, minced
1 cup low fat beef broth
1 tablespoon apple cider vinegar

Directions

1. Mix together all the rub ingredients in a small bowl.
2. Rub the spice mix all over the pork
3. Place the garlic, onion, beef broth and apple cider vinegar in the slow cooker. Stir a few times to mix well.
4. Add the pork.
5. Set on LOW and cook for 4-6 hours until the pork is cooked through and shred easily with a fork.

Note: pork can be used to make tacos, sandwiches, and salads.

Nutritional Information:
Calories 190, Total Fat 4.3 g, Saturated Fat 1.2 g, Total Carbohydrate 5.4 g, Dietary Fiber 1.1 g, Sugars 0.9 g, Protein 32.8 g

Curried Pork Chops

Serves: 4
9 SmartPoints™

Ingredients:
1 pound boneless pork chops, approximately ¼ inch thick
Cooking spray
1 teaspoon salt
1 teaspoon black pepper
2 ½ cups carrots, sliced
1 cup unsweetened coconut milk
1 ½ tablespoon curry powder
1 teaspoon lime zest
Cooked rice for serving, optional

Directions:
1. Preheat the oven to 450°F and spray an 8x8 or larger baking dish with cooking spray.
2. Season the pork with salt and black pepper.
3. Place the pork and the sliced carrots in the baking dish, spreading them out into as even a layer as possible.
4. In a bowl, combine the coconut milk, curry powder, and lime zest. Mix well and pour over the pork.
5. Place the baking dish in the oven and bake for 25-30 minutes, or until the pork is cooked through and the carrots are tender.
6. Remove from the oven and let it rest for several minutes before serving.
7. Serve with cooked rice, if desired.

Nutritional Information:
Calories 367, Total Fat 20.1 g, Saturated Fat 7.5 g, Total Carbohydrate 9.9 g, Dietary Fiber 2.2 g, Sugars 3.4 g, Protein 34.9 g

Spicy Pineapple Pork

Serves: 4
8 SmartPoints™

Ingredients:
1 pound cooked pork, shredded
1 tablespoon vegetable oil or cooking spray
3 cups broccoli florets
1 teaspoon salt
1 teaspoon black pepper
2 cups medium heat tomato salsa, fresh or jarred
2 cups fresh pineapple chunks
¼ cup fresh orange juice (or other citrus juice of choice)
Fresh cilantro for serving (optional)
Cooked rice for serving (optional)

Directions:
1. Heat the vegetable oil or cooking spray in a large skillet over medium heat.
2. Add the broccoli and sauté for 5-7 minutes, or until crisp tender.
3. Add the shredded pork to the skillet and season with salt and black pepper.
4. Next, add the salsa, pineapple chunks, and orange juice. Mix well.
5. Increase the heat to medium high until the liquid comes to a low boil.
6. Reduce the heat to low, cover, and simmer for 5-7 minutes, or until heated through.
7. Remove from the heat and serve with cooked rice and cilantro, if desired.

Nutritional Information:
Calories 328, Total Fat 10.3 g, Saturated Fat 2.5 g, Total Carbohydrate 22.7 g, Dietary Fiber 5.0 g, Sugars 9.4 g, Protein 37.4 g

Breaded Veal Cutlets

Serves 4
6 SmartPoints™

Ingredients
1 pound veal cutlets, trimmed

Cooking spray
1/2 cup dry whole-wheat breadcrumbs
1/2 teaspoon paprika
1/2 teaspoon onion powder
1/2 teaspoon salt and black pepper
4 teaspoons canola oil
1 large egg white
4 teaspoons cornstarch

Directions
1. Pound the veal cutlet if needed, so they are ½ inch thick.
2. Preheat oven to 400°F. And line a rimmed baking sheet with parchment paper. Spray lightly with cooking spray.
3. Mix breadcrumbs, and spices in a shallow bowl. Add the oil and mix well.
4. Sprinkle cornstarch over the veal cutlets to evenly coat both sides.
5. Beat the egg white until it becomes frothy. Place in a shallow dish.
6. Add the veal cutlets to the egg white. Massage to coat. Add the cutlets one by one to the breadcrumbs and spices mixt. Try to coat as evenly as possible.
7. Arrange the veal cutlets on the baking sheet. Bake in the preheated oven for 15to 18 minutes, until golden and cooked through.

Nutritional Information:
Calories 219, Total Fat 7 g, Saturated Fat 2.7 g, Total Carbohydrate 11.2 g, Dietary Fiber 1.1 g, Sugars 1.7 g, Protein 24.8 g

Cheesy Fajita Casserole

Serves: 4, 5 SmartPoints™

Ingredients:
½ teaspoon salt
1 teaspoon coarse ground black pepper
1 teaspoon cumin
½ teaspoon cayenne powder
½ teaspoon smoked paprika
Cooking spray
1 pound chicken breast tenders
2 cups yellow and green bell peppers, sliced
1 cup red onion, sliced
1 cup stewed tomatoes, chopped, juice included
¾ cup queso fresco cheese, crumbled

Fresh cilantro for garnish (optional)
Directions:
1. Combine the salt, black pepper, cumin, cayenne powder and smoked paprika. Set aside.
2. Preheat the oven to 375°F and spray an 8x8 or larger baking dish with cooking spray.
3. Arrange the chicken tenders in an even layer in the baking dish and season liberally with at least half of the seasoning mixture.
4. Place the bell peppers and onions over the chicken, followed by the stewed tomatoes.
5. Add any remaining seasoning mixture to the top of the peppers and onions.
6. Sprinkle the queso fresco cheese over the top and place the pan in the oven.
7. Bake uncovered for 25-30 minutes, or until the chicken is cooked through.
8. Remove from the oven and let sit for 5 minutes.
9. Serve warm, garnished with fresh cilantro, if desired.

Nutritional Information:
Calories 233, Total Fat 7.7 g, Saturated Fat 3.8 g, Total Carbohydrate 8.7 g, Dietary Fiber 2.0 g, Sugars 1.5 g, Protein 31.4 g

Spiced Pork with Apples

Serves: 6
5 SmartPoints™
Ingredients:
2 (14 ounce) pork tenderloins
Olive oil cooking spray
2 teaspoon 5-spice powder, divided
2 apples, cored and sliced
1 red onion, sliced
Directions:
1. Preheat the oven to 450°F. Remove any excess fat from the pork.
2. Line the baking pan with foil. Spray the foil lightly with olive oil cooking spray. Sprinkle 1 teaspoon 5-spice powder on the pork tenderloins and then place them on the baking pan. Roast the pork for about 20 to 30 minutes, or until it is ready.

3. Meanwhile, spray a non-stick pan with cooking spray and sauté the sliced onion until tender. Add 1 teaspoon 5-spice powder and mix well. Add the apple slices and sauté again until the mixture becomes soft and the onions are cooked. Cut the pork tenderloins into ½-inch slices and top them with the apple and onion mixture. Serve.

Nutritional Information:
Calories 253, Total Fat 9.3 g, Saturated Fat 3.2 g, Total Carbohydrate 9.2 g, Dietary Fiber 1.7 g, Sugars 4.1 g, Protein 31.9 g

Pork Chops with Salsa

Serves: 4
4 SmartPoints™
Ingredients:
4 ounces boneless pork loin chops (lean), trimmed
Cooking spray
⅓ Cup salsa
2 tablespoons lime juice, freshly squeezed
¼ cup fresh cilantro or parsley, chopped
Directions:
1. Place the chops on a flat surface and press each one of them with the palm of your hand to flatten them slightly.
2. Coat a large, nonstick skillet with cooking spray. Place it over high heat until the oil becomes hot. Add the chops to the skillet and cook each side for 1 minute, or until they are colored medium-brown. Reduce the heat to medium-low.
3. Mix the salsa and the fresh lime juice together and pour the mixture over the chops. Simmer, uncovered for about 8 minutes or until the chops are cooked through.
4. Garnish the chops with chopped cilantro or parsley (if desired). Serve.

Nutritional Information:
Calories 184, Total Fat 8.0 g, Saturated Fat 12.0 g, Total Carbohydrate 2.0 g, Sugars 0.6 g, Protein 25.0 g

Italian Steak Rolls

Serves: 4
5 SmartPoints™

Ingredients:
1 pound flank steak, thinly sliced in sheets
¼ cup low fat Italian salad dressing
1 cup red bell pepper, sliced
½ pound asparagus spears, trimmed
1 cup onion, sliced
Cooking spray
1 teaspoon salt
1 teaspoon black pepper
Kitchen twine

Directions:
1. Place the steaks in a bowl and cover them with the Italian salad dressing. Toss to coat. Set aside for 15 minutes.
2. Preheat the oven to 350°F and line a baking sheet with aluminum foil.
3. Remove the meat from the marinade and lay the slices out on a flat surface. Season with salt and black pepper as desired.
4. Place the red bell pepper, asparagus and onion pieces on the center of each piece of meat in equal amounts.
5. Roll up each piece of meat around the vegetables and secure with kitchen twine.
6. Heat the cooking spray in a skillet over medium high.
7. Add the steak rolls to the skillet and sear on all sides.
7. Transfer the steak rolls to the baking sheet. Place it in the oven and bake for 15-20 minutes, or until the meat is cooked through and the vegetables are crisp tender.
8. Remove from the oven and let rest 5 minutes before serving.

Nutritional Information:
Calories 211, Total Fat 8.6 g, Saturated Fat 3.7 g, Total Carbohydrate 7.9 g, Dietary Fiber 1.9 g, Sugars 1.8 g, Protein 24.6 g

Creamy Dijon Chicken

Serves: 4
3 SmartPoints™

Ingredients:
1 pound boneless, skinless chicken breasts
1 tablespoon olive oil or cooking spray
1 teaspoon salt
1 teaspoon white pepper
1 teaspoon fresh thyme
¼ cup Dijon mustard
½ cup low fat milk
2 cloves garlic, crushed and minced
4 cups fresh spinach, torn

Directions:
1. Heat the olive oil in a skillet over medium heat.
2. Using a meat mallet, pound the chicken until it reaches a thickness of approximately ¼ inch.
3. Season the chicken with salt, white pepper and fresh thyme. Add the chicken to the skillet and cook for 3-4 minutes per side.
4. Combine the Dijon mustard, milk, and garlic.
5. Add the Dijon mixture to the skillet and cook for 1-2 minutes.
6. Add the spinach and cook an additional 4-5 minutes, turning the chicken occasionally, until the chicken is cooked through and the spinach is wilted.
7. Remove from heat and serve warm with favorite accompaniment.

Nutritional Information:
Calories 170, Total Fat 3.2 g, Saturated Fat 0.8 g, Total Carbohydrate 2.6 g, Dietary Fiber 0.7 g, Sugars 1.7 g, Protein 27.6 g

Light Chicken Salad

Serves: 3
4 SmartPoints™

Ingredients:
2 pieces boneless chicken breast
2 celery stalks, finely chopped
1 chicken bouillon cube
¼ onion, chopped

3 tablespoons light mayonnaise
2 tablespoons parsley chopped

Directions:
1. Place the chicken breasts, half of the chopped celery, half the onion, and parsley in a medium saucepan. Cover the ingredients with water. Add the chicken bouillon cube, and cover with a lid.
2. Cook on medium heat for about 15 to 20 minutes, or until the chicken has cooked through. Remove the chicken from the heat and let it cool. Reserve the chicken broth.
3. Dice the chicken and place it in a bowl. Add the remaining celery, onions, and the mayonnaise. Add ⅛ cup of the chicken broth you had reserved, and mix well. Add more if the chicken looks dry. Serve on lettuce, as a lettuce wrap, or on bread.

Nutritional Information:
Calories 169, Total Fat 5.3 g, Saturated Fat 2.8 g, Total Carbohydrate 4.1 g, Dietary Fiber 1.0 g, Sugars 1.1 g, Protein 25.4 g

Turkey Mac with Jalapenos

Serves: 8, 8 SmartPoints™

Ingredients:
2 teaspoon chili powder
1 teaspoon garlic powder
1 teaspoon ground coriander
1 teaspoon onion powder
1 teaspoon cumin
¼ teaspoon salt
1 tablespoon olive oil
1 pound ground turkey
3 cups beef broth
1 (10 ounce) can tomatoes with green chilies, diced
2 cups dry whole wheat elbow pasta
½ cup low fat milk
4 ounces cream cheese
1 cup cheddar cheese, shredded
½ cup pickled jalapenos, chopped

Directions:
1. In a small bowl, mix together the chili powder, garlic powder, ground coriander, onion powder, chili powder, cumin, and salt.

2. In a medium saucepan, heat the olive oil on medium-high. Add the turkey and cook until it turns color. Add the spices, mix them in, and allow the mixture to cook for a further 1 or 2 minutes. Stir in the beef broth, diced tomatoes, and dry pasta. Cover the pot and cook for about 8 to 10 minutes.
3. Before the pasta finish cooking, poor the milk in a pot and place it over low heat. When the milk is warm and steamy, mix in the cheese cream until it melts. The shredded cheese can then be added to the milk. Stir until it melts.
4. Empty the cheese sauce into the pasta blend and mix until the pasta is equally covered. Blend in the pickled jalapenos. Give it a taste and add more salt if necessary. Serve hot.

Nutritional Information:
Calories 322, Total Fat 15.0 g, Saturated Fat 4.8 g, Total Carbohydrate 20.3 g, Dietary Fiber 4.0 g, Sugars 11.2 g, Protein 20.0 g

Grilled Chicken Salad

Serves: 4
6 SmartPoints™
Ingredients:
¼ cup mayonnaise (low-fat)
1 teaspoon curry powder
2 teaspoons water
4 ounces or 1 cup rotisserie chicken, preferably lemon herb flavor, chopped
¾ cup apple, chopped
⅓ Cup celery, diced
3 tablespoons raisins
⅛ Teaspoon salt
Directions:
1. In a medium-sized bowl, combine the mayonnaise, curry powder, and water. Stir with a whisk until well blended.
2. Add the chopped chicken, celery, raisins, chopped apple, and salt. Stir the ingredients so they get combined well. Cover the salad and chill in the fridge. Serve in a lettuce wrap, with bread, or on its own.

Nutritional Information:
Calories 222, Total Fat 5.4 g, Saturated Fat 2.1 g, Total Carbohydrate 26.9 g, Dietary Fiber 2.5 g, Sugars 8.1 g, Protein 23.0 g

Delicious Chicken Salad

Serves: 4
4 SmartPoints™
Ingredients:
2 ½ cups chicken, cooked and chopped
3 stalks celery, chopped
1 cup apple, chopped
¼ cup cranberries, dried
½ cup plain Greek yogurt (nonfat)
2 tablespoons Hellman's mayonnaise, light
2 teaspoons lemon juice
Salt and pepper to taste
<u>Optional</u>:
2 tablespoons fresh parsley, chopped
Directions:
1. In a large bowl, mix the chicken, celery, apple, and dried cranberries. Stir the ingredients and combine them well.
2. In a small bowl, mix the yogurt, mayonnaise, and lemon juice. Add the mixture to the chicken mixture and mix well. Stir in the chopped parsley, if using. Add salt and pepper to taste.
3. Serve on whole grain crackers, rice, pita bread, or make a wrap.

Nutritional Information:
Calories 220 Total Fat 5.0 g, Saturated Fat 1.1 g, Total Carbohydrate 13.0 g, Dietary Fiber 2.0 g, Sugars 7.1 g, Protein 28.0 g

Raspberry Balsamic Chicken

Serves: 3
5 SmartPoints™
Ingredients:
3 pieces boneless skinless chicken breast
¼ cup all-purpose flour
Cooking spray
⅔ Cup chicken broth (low fat)
½ cup raspberry preserve (low sugar)
1 ½ teaspoons cornstarch
1 ½ tablespoons balsamic vinegar
Salt and black pepper to taste
Directions:

1. Cut the boneless and skinless chicken breast into bite-sized pieces. (You may also pound them into thin cutlets to cook through easily.) Season the chicken with salt and black pepper to taste. Dredge the chicken pieces in the flour, and shake off any excess.
2. Heat a non-stick skillet over medium heat and coat it with spray. Cook the chicken for about 15 minutes, turning halfway through so both sides can cook well. Remove the cooked chicken from the skillet.
3. Mix the chicken broth, raspberry preserves, and cornstarch in the skillet over medium heat. Stir in the balsamic vinegar. Add chicken back to the pan. Cook for about 10 minutes, turning halfway through.

Nutritional Information:
Calories 229, Total Fat 4. 6 g, Saturated Fat 0.8 g, Total Carbohydrate 21.8 g, Dietary Fiber 0.7 g, Sugars 15.0 g, Protein 24.5 g

Final Words

Thank for making it through to the end of *this book*. Let's hope it was informative and able to provide you with all of the tools you need to achieve your weight loss goals.

Natasha Hayward

Made in the USA
Middletown, DE
06 July 2019